Adult-Gerontology Acute Care NP Study Guide 2021-2022

2021-2022

New Outline + 450 Questions and Answer Explanations for the Acute Care Nurse Practitioner Exam (Includes 3 Full-length Practice Tests)

ISBN (paperback): 978-1-989726-63-1

Newstone Test Prep

Table of Contents

Introduction

Gerontology is the study of the biological, sociocultural, psychological and cognitive dimensions of aging. It is different from geriatrics in that geriatrics focuses on the management of diseases in the elderly. An adult-gerontology nurse practitioner (AGNP) is an advanced practice registered nurse who is trained to manage patients from adolescence into adulthood and then into their old age. Unlike registered nurses, an adult-gerontology nurse practitioner can prescribe drugs, request and interpret laboratory tests and write and implement treatment plans for patients.

There are two kinds of AGNPs: adult-gerontology acute care nurse practitioners (AG-ACNPs) and adult-gerontology primary care nurse practitioners (AG-PCNPs). This study guide was created specifically to prepare you to become an AG-ACNP. These professionals provide health education and counseling on disease prevention, lifestyle modification and management of chronic diseases and disabilities. Although these nurses are trained to work in a broad range of settings like clinics, hospitals, ambulatory care centers and others, community-based care is their primary responsibility.

Who Is an AG-ACNP?

An AG-ACNP specializes in providing care to adolescents and adults who have an acute illness, episodic disease or exacerbated terminal or chronic disease. These nurses are trained to prescribe drugs, request and interpret diagnostic tests and create full medical treatment plans for their patients. They may specialize in subunits like trauma, oncology, surgery, critical care and cardiopulmonary, and they are found in emergency rooms, ICUs and other settings that offer acute care. AG-ACNPs are key players in the health-care system in the United States, helping to mitigate the effects of a physician shortage. The functions of an AG-ACNP include:

Acute health management – This is a broad role that includes rapid assessment and emergency resuscitation of acute patients, interventions like intubation and insertion of intravenous lines, requests for and interpretation of diagnostic tests, commencement of pharmacological therapies, creation of treatment plans and management of patients' pain.

Health advocacy – Apart from providing health care to acutely ill patients, the AG-ACNP also acts as a health advocate for patients in terms of providing for physical, psychological, biological, sociocultural and religious needs. For example, an AG-ACNP is interested not only in administering adequate pain relief to a Muslim patient with a femoral fracture secondary to a road traffic accident but also in providing an environment that is conducive for the patient's religious rites.

Therapeutic communication – Just like all health care personnel, the AG-ACNP uses therapeutic communication skills to attend to patients' needs. AG-ACNPs treat vulnerable patients, and they must convey and receive information with empathy and professionalism.

Health education – AG-ACNPs are responsible for educating patients and their caregivers on the management, progression and possible complications of diseases. They are also responsible for providing important information that can help patients and their caregivers make informed decisions on medical treatment and medicolegal situations.

Mentorship and tutorials – Because AG-ACNPs are nursing professionals with advanced training, they are responsible for mentoring junior colleagues like registered nurses, licensed practitioner nurses, nursing assistants and others.

Requirements to Become an Adult-Gerontology Acute Care Nurse Practitioner

1. **An undergraduate degree program in nursing** – This includes a two-year diploma or associate degree program in nursing or a four-year baccalaureate program in nursing. The four-year baccalaureate program is preferable.

2. **Licensure as a registered nurse** – This involves passing the NCLEX-RN exams (National Council Licensure Examination for Registered Nurses). The NCLEX-RN exams test the skills and knowledge of entry-level nurses to determine whether a nurse is skilled enough to be licensed for practice. The test questions are administered by the NCSBN on behalf of the member boards. These member boards include nursing boards in the 10 provinces in Canada, the 50 states in America, the District of Columbia and four US territories (American Samoa, Northern Mariana Islands, Guam and the US Virgin Islands).

3. **Master of science degree or doctoral degree in nursing** – These programs take at least a year to complete. Most degrees can be completed online, and most allow practicing registered nurses with a bachelor of science degree to continue working. A master's or doctoral degree is a requirement to become a nurse practitioner and a requirement for nurses who wish to become Advanced Practice Registered Nurses (APRNs).

4. **Work experience** – To qualify for the AG-ACNP licensing exam, you are expected to have prior professional experience as a registered nurse or nurse practitioner. This is usually measured as at least 500 to 600 hours of faculty-supervised clinical rotations.

Licensing and Certification

Certification as an AG-ACNP can be obtained from either the American Association of Critical-Care Nurses or the American Nurses Credentialing Center. This book reviews the application process and test offered by the American Association of Critical-Care Nurses.

Certification by the American Nurses Credentialing Center (ANCC)

The ANCC awards the Adult-Gerontology Acute Care Nurse Practitioner Board Certified Credential (ACNP-BC) to successful candidates. The board certification exam assesses the clinical skills and knowledge of entry-level nurse practitioners according to the APRN model of regulation, which is licensure, accreditation, certification and education. This credential is valid for up to five years and can be renewed according to the requirements of the licensing body.

Eligibility requirements for the ACNP-BC include a valid and active RN license in the United States or the legal equivalent from another country and a master's or doctoral degree from an accredited AG-ACNP program. Such accreditation must be either from the Commission on Collegiate Nursing Education (CCNE) or Accreditation Commission for Education in Nursing (ACEN). Also required are at least 500 hours of faculty-supervised clinical hours and other separate graduate-level courses in advanced health assessment, advanced physiology/pathophysiology and advanced pharmacology.

Career Options for an AG-ACNP

AG-ACNPs can work inside or outside a hospital setting.

Career options in hospital settings – AG-ACNPs work in emergency rooms, intensive care units, burn and trauma centers, specialty labs, acute and subacute care wards and specialty clinics.

Career options outside hospital settings – AG-ACNPs work in ambulatory care facilities, urgent care centers, rehabilitation centers, hospice care centers and palliative care centers.

Pay

In the nursing field, nursing practitioners usually earn the highest salary. According to the Bureau of Labor Statistics, AG-ACNPs earn an average of about $101,260 a year. Salaries can range from $70,540 to $135,800 a year, depending on work experience, location and type of employer.

1. Location – AG-ACNPs in rural areas are paid less than their colleagues in urban areas. According to the Bureau of Labor Statistics, the top-paying states for nurse practitioners in 2015 were:

California – $120,930 average annual salary

Alaska – $117,080 annual average salary

Hawaii – $114,220 average annual salary

Massachusetts – $112,860 average annual salary

Oregon – $111,210 average annual salary

Be aware that areas with higher salaries may have a higher cost of living.

2. Type of facility – Health workers in federal facilities earn considerably more than their colleagues in private establishments. However, getting jobs in federal facilities is competitive because of the limited spaces available.

3. Experience – Experience is a key determinant in the amount of salary a person earns. For example, in 2015, the American Association of Nurse Practitioners did a national nurse practitioner compensation survey of 25,000 nurses across the country and discovered these trends in salary:

0–5 years' experience: $92,410 average annual salary

6–10 years: $99,221 average annual salary

11–15 years: $101,364 average annual salary

16–20 years: $105,507 average annual salary

21 years and above: $106,669 average annual salary

Pros and Cons of Becoming an Adult-Gerontology Acute Care Nurse Practitioner

It is good to evaluate the pros and cons of choosing to become an AG-ACNP.

Pros

1. **Humanitarian service** – Like other health-related services, nurses provide direct service to humans. It can be deeply rewarding to use your skills, time and expertise to save a life.

2. **Excitement** – AG-ACNPs work in settings that provide acute care to emergency and trauma patients.

3. **Job security** – The demand for nurse practitioners is projected to increase dramatically in the coming years as baby boomers age, the number of physicians declines and the demand for health-care professionals in rural areas increases.

Cons

1. **Long hours** – Nurse practitioners work long hours that may include 12-hour shifts, night shifts and call duties. Nurses work every day of the week, all year round, on weekends, during summer holidays and on national holidays.

2. **Emotional and physical burnout** – Like other health-care workers, nurses are vulnerable to emotional and physical burnout. This is because providing care to sick people is demanding. Nursing also involves a lot of physical activity, such as carrying, lifting and pushing. Also, nurses provide emotional support and compassion to all their patients, including the difficult ones. Nurses have to deal with the loss of their patients, even after putting in maximum effort to save their lives. Additionally, Nurses have to make split-second decisions in critical cases and emergencies.

3. **Exposure to biohazards** – Nurses are vulnerable to biohazards like needleprick injuries, infected aerosols, infected contact surfaces and radiation. Biohazards are serious and can be life-threatening.

Traits of a successful AG-ACNP

1. **Ability to work in a high-pressure environment** – An AG-ACNP is expected to quickly and accurately assess the condition of critical patients, make clinical decisions and convey information to the patient and caregivers. Nurse practitioners are expected to perform all these tasks in a tense, high-pressure environment while remaining calm and professional.

2. **Decision making** – An AG-ACNP must make quick and accurate decisions on a daily basis.

3. **Leadership and administration** – An AG-ACNP is responsible for assessing patients and creating treatment plans for them. The nurse practitioner is the head of the nursing team, and in cases when there is no physician, he or she is also the head of the medical team. Note that this means the nurse practitioner may be held responsible for unfavorable outcomes.

4. **Empathy** – An AG-ACNP should have empathy for both patients and caregivers, using therapeutic communication techniques to convey and receive information.

5. **Team player** – A successful AG-ACNP is a team player and collaborator who knows how to function with other members of the health team.

Chapter 1: The ACNPC-AG Exam

What Is the ACNPC-AG Exam?

The Acute Care Nurse Practitioner - Adult-Gerontology Certification Exam is administered by the AACN. This exam is given to new graduate nurse practitioners who wish to specialize in the care of acutely ill adolescents and adults. By providing a standardized psychometric exam that assesses the ability of candidates to perform safely and efficiently as entry-level AG-ACNPs, the exam protects the public from unqualified professionals.

The AACN is guided by a set of values: leadership, integrity, commitment to excellence, stewardship and promotion of research-based credentialing programs. Over the years, the AACN has certified approximately 125,000 nurses in the United States.

The ACNPC-AG exam is based on a job analysis that is conducted every five years to ensure that the methods used to assess the skills and knowledge of entry-level AG-ACNPs are within the scope of the study of practice. The certification exam meets the criteria for the APRN Consensus Model and the NCSBN Criteria for APRN Certification Programs.

Eligibility Requirements

Eligibility requirements for the ACNPC-AG exam are in keeping with the criteria set by the APRN and NCSBN. Because of this, state boards of nursing can use the exam results to determine eligibility for an APRN licensure. Registered nurses who are preparing to start a master's program and want AACN certification must ensure that their graduate programs comply with both state and national standards. The eligibility requirements include:

1. Licensure – You are expected to have a current and unencumbered RN or APRN license from the United States. An unencumbered license is required to be free from formal discipline and sanctions by the board of nursing in the state where you are practicing. The license must also not have any limitations on your nursing practice. These limitations include but are not limited to direct supervision of the nursing practice, limitations on drug administration and/or exclusions on practice areas. If limitations are placed on the RN/APRN license, you must inform the AACN Certification Corporation within 30 days.

Nurses with encumbered licenses may be eligible for conditional certification, pending the review of their licenses. Conditional certification is temporary and granted to nurses seeking APRN certification with a provision/condition placed on their RB/APRN licenses. Unconditional status will be converted to active status when the provision/condition is removed and the license becomes unencumbered. If the state board of nursing suspends or revokes the nurse's license, the conditional certification will then also be revoked.

2. Education – You are expected to complete a graduate-level advanced practice education program that satisfies the following criteria:

1. The program is administered in a college that awards CCNE- or ACEN-accredited master's degrees or higher in nursing that focus on training for AD-ACNP. The program must also have in-depth training on how to care for all adults (i.e., young adults, older adults and the elderly).

2. The program is in full compliance with the National Taskforce Criteria for Evaluation of Nurse Practitioner Programs.

3. Direct and indirect clinical supervision must comply with AACN and other accreditation guidelines.

4. The curriculum must provide practical and theoretical training on biological, behavioral, medical and nursing sciences including advanced courses in pathophysiology, pharmacology and physical assessment. The curriculum must also provide training on the legal, ethical and professional responsibilities of the AG-ACNP, as well as supervised clinical practice that is relevant to the specialty of acute care.

5. The curriculum must be consistent with the competencies of AG-ACNP practice and must have at least 500 hours of mandatory clinical supervision. Supervised clinical hours must focus on direct care of acutely ill gerontology patients in the United States.

6. Official transcripts for all coursework must be sent to the AACN either via the school's email or in a sealed envelope from the school.

Pass Rates

The AACN published data on the pass rates for the past three years. The itemized data includes the total number of candidates tested for the year, first-time pass rates for the year, the total number of certificates, renewed certificates and the total number of failed and new certificates.

Pass Rates for the ACNPC-AG from 2017-2019

Year	Number of Candidates Tested	First-Time Pass Rate	Total Certifications	Renewed	Total Failed	New Certificants
2017	554	73.0%	899	N/A	N/A	N/A
2018	562	80.4%	1,296	40	159	344
2019	546	81.4%	1,696	61	141	405

How to Register for the ACNPC-AG Exam

1. Application – You can register for the exam either by filling out the application online or by completing a paper application.

Online Application – You can register on the AACN website at www.aacn.org/certification. Click on the **Get Certified** tab to register for a computer-based exam.

To register, you are expected to have:

1. A current and unencumbered RN/APRN license number and expiration date.

2. A credit card, which can be a Visa, MasterCard, Discover Card or American Express.

3. Scanned copies of your original, final transcripts for all graduate-level courses. These transcripts must show the degrees and the dates upon which they were conferred. Electronic transcripts can be emailed directly from the school. Mailed transcripts can be sent to the AACN directly from the school.

4. An Educational Eligibility Form that is completed by the program director. This form should be uploaded to the Program Director Portal.

Paper Application – Submit all of the following in a signed and sealed envelope that is mailed to the AACN:

1. Original and final transcripts for all graduate-level work. These transcripts must show the degrees and the dates upon which they were conferred. Electronic transcripts can be emailed directly from the school. Mailed transcripts can be sent to the AACN directly from the school.

2. An Educational Eligibility Form that is completed by the director of the ACNP program.

3. An Honor Statement Form that you complete and sign.

4. Evidence of payment via credit card, check or money order.

   You must fill out the application form with your legal name that matches the name on your photo ID, certificate and license.

2. Notification – After applying for the exam with the relevant forms and making payment, you will receive an email confirming reception of the application and notifying you that the application has been sent to a certified specialist for evaluation. This evaluation typically takes from one to four weeks. The time frame depends on whether the AANC contacts your school for more information to verify your eligibility.

3. Approval – Next, you will receive an email of approval to take the exam, along with a scheduling email from PSI, the AACN's testing service provider. This scheduling email will be sent about five to 10 days after the confirmation email, within two weeks of online registration and within four weeks of paper registration. The email will contain instructions on how to schedule your testing appointment, a toll-free number for clarifications and resolution of issues, your exam number and AACN number and the 90-day period during which you must schedule a date for the exam. If you do not receive the approval and scheduling emails, contact AACN's customer care.

4. Schedule the exam – Schedule your preferred date and time of examination within the 90-day testing window as soon as possible. PSI centers administer tests twice a day, at 9 a.m. and 1:30 p.m., Monday through Friday. Saturday appointments are possible at a few testing centers. Visit www.goAMP.com to choose a testing center or schedule an appointment by phone. To schedule an exam, you must provide the test ID number written both on your confirmation postcard and in your confirmation email. After scheduling, a confirmation email will be sent to you with your scheduled date and time. Unscheduled candidates will *not* be allowed into the testing center.

Exams are offered either on a computer or using standard pencil-and-paper format. Results of computer exams are offered on-site as soon as the test is completed, while results of the paper-and-pencil format are emailed about six to eight weeks after the date you took the test. Successful candidates are emailed their certificates about one to two weeks after the test results are received.

Testing is done in more than 300 PSI sites in the United States. Candidates are scheduled on a first-come, first-served basis, so it is important to schedule an appointment as soon as you are ready to test. After receiving the notification email from PSI, make sure you confirm the name and exam type because these cannot be changed at the exam center. If there are discrepancies in the information provided, contact AACN customer care as soon as possible.

Application Fees

As stated earlier, payment can be made via credit card for online applications, and also via check or money order for paper applications. Candidates considered ineligible and who are disqualified from taking the exam will have the exam fees refunded, minus a $15 charge for returned checks.

ACNPC-AG Application Fees

Designation	AACN Member	Nonmember
Computer-based exam	$260	$370
Retake exam	$200	$305
Renewal by exam	$200	$305

ACNPC-AG Certification Renewal

The ACNPC-AG certificate is valid for five years. The certification period starts from the first day of the month when the ACNPC-AG exam was passed and ends five years later. ACNP-AGs are emailed renewal notifications four months before their ACNPC-AG renewal date. Nursing practitioners (NPs) are responsible for renewing their certification, whether they get the notification emails or not.

Renewal is necessary to encourage continued learning and competence. This continued learning is measured by any of the following criteria:

1. Practice hours and continuing education, including pharmacology continuing education
2. Practice hours, pharmacology continuing education and passing the certification exam
3. Continuing education, including pharmacology continuing education and passing the certification exam.

There are certain limitations to the components of the renewal options.

1. Limitations to **continuing education** are based on the quality of the educational content, its relevance to practice and the NP's ability to choose materials that are important to individual practice and educational needs.
2. Limitations to the **practice hours** are based on the quality of the practice environment and available learning opportunities.
3. Limitations to the **certification exam** are based on the exam's ability to test the AG-ACNP's new competencies.

To reduce these limitations, the AANC requires that multiple criteria are met.

Eligibility

AG-ACNPs must renew their certification before the expiration date. To do so, they have to satisfy current ACNPC-AG eligibility requirements and pass the certification exam.

To be eligible to take the renewal exam, you are required to have a current and unencumbered RN/APRN license.

Options for renewal include:

- **Option 1** – 1,000 practice hours and 150 CE points
- **Option 2** – 1,000 practice hours, 25 pharmacology CE points and exam
- **Option 3** – 50 CE points and exam.

What to Expect on the Exam Day

1. Check in – You must arrive at the designated testing center at least 30 minutes before your scheduled time. This is to enable you to check in, find your seat and be comfortably settled before the exam begins. If you arrive more than 15 minutes after the exam, you will not be allowed to test. PSI sites are typically located in H&R Block offices. On arrival, be on the lookout for signs that indicate the check-in location for the testing center. Items that are prohibited from the testing center include reference materials like books, papers and dictionaries; personal items like purses, headwear, hoodies, veils, coats, briefcases and others. PSI, the AACN and H&R Block will not take responsibility for missing or stolen items, so any personal items should be left at home or in your vehicle.

2. Identification – Two types of ID are required for identification: the primary and secondary ID. The primary ID should be current, issued by a government agency and include a signature and a photograph. Acceptable primary IDs include a driver's license, state ID card, passport and military ID card. The secondary ID must have your signature and legal name. Examples are a credit card, membership card/check cashing card,

Social Security card or employment/student ID card. Note that temporary means of identification are usually not accepted at exam centers.

3. Seating arrangements – After checking in, you will be directed to your designated testing carrel. If you scheduled a computer exam, you will be given a computer and a chair. The computer software will instruct you to enter your AACN custom ID number. Your photograph will be captured by the computer to show on your score report.

If you scheduled a paper-and-pencil test, you will be given a booklet and a Scantron form.

You should wear comfortable clothing that suits the temperature of the exam room. If the weather is unfavorable, the management team at PSI will decide if the exam should be canceled. If the exam is canceled, you will be informed of the rescheduled dates and/or reapplication process.

Taking the Computer-Based Exam (CBT)

The CBT exam is a multiple-choice exam. The number of correct questions determines your score.

1. Practice exam – You will first be given a practice exam to familiarize yourself with the CBT software interface. The time used for the practice exam is not added to your timed exam.

2. Timed exam – This is the actual exam. Instructions for taking the exam will appear on-screen. There is a time limit for this exam, and the software will log you out as soon as that time limit has been exceeded. Be sure to answer all questions quickly and efficiently.

3. How to answer the test questions – The software displays only one question at a time. Use the mouse to click the correct answer in the lower-left section of the screen. You can change your answers as much as you want. To move to the next test item, click on the forward arrow. To move back to the previous test item, click on the backward arrow.

You can leave a test item unanswered and return to it later. To answer the easier questions first, then return to the difficult ones when time permits, bookmark a test item. Just click on the blank square to the right of the **Time** button. Remember to answer all questions because there is no penalty for guessing.

4. Exam protocol – You are not allowed to ask questions about the content of the exam. You will be given scratch paper if you need to make notes during the exam. These scratch notes must be returned at the end of the exam, along with any question papers and written materials given to you for the exam. You can contest any item by clicking on the **Comment** button that is located on the left of the **Time** button. A dialogue box will open, and you can enter your comments.

Breaks are part of the timed exam. You can ask for a break as often as you wish, but remember that no extra time will be given. You are not allowed to eat, drink or smoke during the exam. You cannot leave your seat without permission. If you finish the exam before the time is over, you can click on the **Exit** button on the screen.

Taking the Paper-and-Pencil Exam

The paper-and-pencil exam is also multiple choice. This means that the number of correct questions determines your score. There are no practice questions in the paper-and-pencil format.

1. How to answer the test items – Use the pencil provided to shade in your answers on the Scantron sheet. Do not make stray marks on your answer sheet. Answer easy questions and return to the difficult ones when time permits. Remember to answer all questions because there is no penalty for guessing.

2. Exam protocol – You are not allowed to ask questions about the content of the exam. You will be given scratch paper if you need to make notes during the exam. These scratch notes must be returned at the end of the exam, along with all question papers and written materials given to you for the exam. You can comment on the test items in the designated area of the Scantron sheet. Do so by writing the item number and any comments in the blank box.

Breaks are part of the timed exam. You can ask for a break as often as you wish, but remember that no extra time will be given. You are not allowed to eat, drink or smoke during the exam. You cannot leave your seat without permission. If you finish the exam before the time is over, you can submit your Scantron sheet, question paper and other materials given to you for the exam.

Getting Test Results

After the exam, you will be asked to complete a short evaluation of your testing experience. The results of a CBT-based test will be provided upon completion of the exam. For a paper-and-pencil test, results will be sent six to eight weeks after the exam. Successful candidates will be mailed their certificates one to two weeks after they receive their results.

Retake Policies

If you do not pass the exam, you can reapply to the AACN Certification Corporation for a retest. Retake candidates are offered a discounted retest fee as long as the prior exam was taken within the most recent 90-day window. You can take the same certification exam up to four times in 12 months. After 12 months, you are required to sign a new honor statement. You may apply for a retest on the AACN website or by mailing a paper application.

Test Accommodation Requirements

Accommodation is available for candidates with disabilities covered by the Americans with Disabilities Act (ADA). To receive these accommodations, candidates are expected to complete the Request for Accommodations Form and the Documentation of Disability-Related Needs Form. The Documentation of Disability-Related Needs Form must be completed by a physician, psychologist, education professional or psychiatrist. These forms must be filled out and submitted at least two to three weeks before the scheduled exam.

Exam Rules, Regulations and Sanctions

The following are prohibited in the ACNPC-AG Certification Exam:

1. Unauthorized admission into the exam hall
2. Causing a disturbance or being abusive or uncooperative
3. Bringing electronic devices like cellular/smartphones, palm computers, calculators, pagers, alarms and other signaling devices into the exam hall
4. Bringing notes or other reference materials into the testing center
5. Attempting to record the test questions
6. Attempting to take the exam on behalf of someone else
7. Giving or receiving help during the exam
8. Leaving the test center during the exam without seeking express permission.

All these can warrant dismissal from the exam by the proctor. Dismissal will result in a nullification of your exam score. Exam fees will not be refunded. The AACN will review the evidence of misconduct to determine if you are eligible for a retake. If granted a retake, you are required to begin a new application and must pay the application fees again.

<u>Failure to report for an exam</u> – If you do not appear for your scheduled exam, you can reapply to take the exam. If you do not reapply within a year's time, you are required to pay a reactivation fee that is equivalent to a retest fee. If you reapply after a year, you must start the application process over again and pay a retest fee

<u>Misuse/disclosure of exam content</u> – If you remove or attempt to remove materials from the testing center, or receive, discuss, disclose, reproduce, distribute, display or misuse a test question or any part of a test question from a certification exam by written, electronic, oral or other form of communication, you will be subject to legal action and monetary damages.

Denial of Certification

The AACN Certification Corporation has the right to deny certification for reasons such as:

1. Violating any rules of the exam
2. Falsifying certification exam application
3. Falsifying any information provided to the AACN Certification Corporation
4. Inability to meet eligibility requirements
5. Inability to pay fees
6. Inability to meet deadlines
7. Inability to respond to or pass an audit
8. Misuse of certification status and credentials
9. Cheating during the exam
10. Sharing exam contents.

If you are denied certification, you will be prohibited from reapplying for the exam for three years. The AACN can also take other disciplinary actions, like notifying your employer and the state board of nursing.

Revocation of Certificate

The AACN Certification Corporation has the right to revoke certification for reasons such as:

1. Falsifying a certification exam application or renewal application
2. Falsifying any information provided to the AACN Certification Corporation
3. Inability to meet/maintain eligibility requirements
4. Inability to pay fees
5. Inability to meet deadlines
6. Inability to respond to or pass an audit

7. Misrepresenting and misusing certification status
8. Conviction of a felony
9. Cheating in the exam
10. Sharing exam contents.

If your certificate is revoked, you may not reapply for any AACN certification exam for three years. Notification may be sent to your employer and the state board of nursing.

Review and Appeal of Certificate Eligibility

You can request a review of eligibility within 45 days of receiving notification of denial. The written request should justify your eligibility for the certification program and contain information supporting your request for reinstatement. Review requests should be received within 30 days of your being notified of the revocation or expiration of your certification. The Internal Review Panel will review the documentation and decide within 30 days.

Appeal of Eligibility, Exam and Renewal Determination

If you believe you were unjustly denied eligibility for an exam or renewal of certification, or if you challenge the results of an exam, you can email a request for reconsideration of the decision. This appeal must be made within 45 days of receipt of the adverse decision and must contain convincing evidence that the decision was unjust. The appeal must also indicate the specific relief requested.

Appeals are addressed by the AACN Certification Corporation Appeals Panel, which is composed of expert peer volunteers. The appeals panel will review the documentation provided and render a decision within 30 days of the date of appeal. The decision of the appeals panel is final and will be sent to you via email.

Exam Structure

The ACNPC-AG exam is a three-and-a-half-hour exam and consists of 175 multiple-choice items. Out of those 175 items, 150 are scored. The remaining 25 items are used to gain insight into statistical data for future exams. Seventy-three percent (73%) of the items are used to test clinical judgment related to nursing care of adult-gerontology patients. The remaining items are used to test non-clinical judgment knowledge and focus on life span.

Passing Standard

The Modified-Angoff is a standard-setting and criterion-referenced process used to set the cut score/passing point standard for an exam. This cut score/passing point is determined by a board of experts in the test's subject matter and an exam development committee (EDC) that reviews all the exam questions and assesses the expected basic level of theoretical and practical knowledge. The cut score/passing point is then based on the panel's standards of difficulty for the test questions. The panel, along with a psychometrician, creates and suggests the cut score, which is then approved by the AACN Certification Corporation.

The aim of the cut score is to assess individuals who possess the standard level of theoretical and practical knowledge. As such, individuals who meet the requirements of the exams have the required amount of knowledge. The cut score is not measured in percentages. It is measured in numbers that change over time, depending on the values from very recent job analyses. The cut score can also change when the exam forms are changed periodically and balanced for difficulty.

Candidate Performance Report

In the performance report, you are provided with the number of questions you answered correctly in each content area. This is to help you assess your level of performance in each content area and to identify your areas of weakness. The questions test not only your knowledge but also your ability to apply that knowledge in carrying out specific skills and abilities required of acute care nurses. Because this exam assesses your knowledge in all areas, you can score high in some areas and still fail the exam. Be aware that the cut score/passing point is not the same as the passing rate.

Tips on How to Pass the ACNP-AG Exam

Passing the ACNP-AG exam requires a combination of preparation, organization and mental attitude. Adequate preparation has a lot to do with the type of resource materials you prepare with, the amount of time you spend preparing and how much information you retain.

How to choose the right resource material

Here are a few things to consider before choosing study material for your exams:

1. **Relevance** – Your study material should be relevant to the exam. To increase your chances of selecting relevant study material, ask for recommendations from tutors, colleagues and peers who have passed the exams.

2. **Revised** – The AACN reviews the ACNP-AG exams every five years. Therefore, your study material should be current, updated and revised to reflect AACN standards.

3. **Cost** – Beware of outrageously expensive materials. There are excellent study resources that are reasonably priced.

4. **Highlights** – Your study material should give highlights on the distribution of test questions and emphasize priority areas to focus on. Focused concentration is a characteristic of effective studying. The right study material should help you narrow your reading to specific, key areas.

5. **Comprehensive rationales** – Your study material should give comprehensive rationales pertaining to test questions and their answers. This fine-tunes your critical thinking and helps you identify subtle distinctions that are important to your exam success.

6. **Organization** – Study materials that break down segments into outlines and sections improve your recall. Conversely, haphazard study materials can slow down your preparation process.

How much time should you spend studying?

It depends on you. There is no one-size-fits-all study duration. But there are a few basic factors that can help you properly prepare a plan of action:

1. **Start early** – Early preparation increases your chances of success because it gives you time to revise and adjust your study plan as needed if you don't find that your first plan is effective.

2. **Have a SMART study goal** – **S**pecific, **M**easurable, **A**chievable, **R**elevant and **T**ime-bound.

For example, let's say you have a study goal to review the 450 questions in this book in a month. This goal has met three requirements of the SMART goal. It is specific, measurable, and time-bound. Now you must assess if the goal is attainable. To do so, determine how many questions you can answer in a day, how much time will be allotted to each study session and if the time allocated is feasible.

3. **Create a study timetable** – A study timetable helps you track your progress and keeps you disciplined and focused. Let's say you assess the feasibility of reviewing this book's 450 questions in one month. Your next step will be to create a detailed study timetable that shows how much time is allocated to each study session.

4. **Choose a suitable study method** – Group studying has its advantages and disadvantages, and so does studying solo. The truth is that neither of the study methods is better than the other. Some candidates study efficiently on their own, some do better

in groups. A good tip is to use both forms of study, devoting more time to your preferred study method.

5. **Enjoy extracurricular activities** – You should factor rest, sleep, breaks and physical activity into your study timetable.

How to improve your recall

Recall is an important aspect of studying. After all, what is the point of reading and reviewing if you cannot recall significant information when you need to? Here are a few tips to improve your recall:

1. *Read actively* – As much as possible, try to engage your mind in the text you are reading. Here are a few tips to help you read actively:

    A. **Read with a focus** – This is where study and resource materials are helpful. By giving you areas to focus on, study materials increase your engagement and concentration.

    B. **Take notes as you read** – Make notes, create mnemonics, questions or a to-do post-reading list. You can also highlight text sections that you want to revisit.

    C. **Take breaks** – Active reading requires focus and effort. Keep study sessions to no more than two to three hours at a time, then take a break. Anything longer, and you may struggle to concentrate.

2. *Study in a group* – Group study is an effective form of active reading. It is great for revising large portions of test questions.

3. *Use mnemonics* – Mnemonics are a great tool for improving your recall. However, they should be used only after understanding the concepts of the topic you read. Mnemonics include but are not limited to acronyms, rhymes, imagery, chunking and use of loci.

4. *Understand first principles* – Nursing is based on the principles of facts, logic and reasoning. Understanding topics from a first-principle basis improves your ability to store and retrieve information. When studying, always try to link the information, building on your knowledge methodically.

5. *Sleep* – Sleep consolidates short-term memory. An adult requires an average of seven to nine hours of sleep a night. Therefore, when you create your study plan, factor in your need to get adequate sleep.

Chapter 2: Content Overview

The AACN Synergy Model for Patient Care is the bedrock of the ACNPC-AG certification program. This model is based on the belief that optimal patient outcomes are achieved through synergistic interaction between the needs of the patient and the competencies of the nurse. This model is highly patient-centered and focused on the nurse's role in providing professional patient care. In this way, nurses are not just health workers. They are also able to see themselves in the context of patients and their outcomes. The two major aspects of the Synergy Model are patient characteristics and nurse Characteristics.

Patient Characteristics

In the Synergy Model, nurses view patients in a holistic manner rather than as compartmentalized body systems. This model encourages nurses to treat each patient and family as unique, identifying their various capacities for health and vulnerability to illness. Every patient comes to the care setting with unique characteristics. The following are the characteristics patients may exhibit based on their position in the health-care continuum:

1. Resiliency – The patient's ability to bounce back to a functional level by using compensatory mechanisms.

2. Participation in decision-making – The level at which the patient and family are involved in decision-making.

3. Predictability – The patient's ability to anticipate the progression of events or illness.

4. Vulnerability – The patient's susceptibility to existing or potential stressors that can severely affect patient outcomes.

5. Resource availability – The fiscal, personal, psychological, technical and social resources that the patient and family/community bring to the scenario.

6. Stability – The patient's capacity to keep equilibrium at a steady state.

7. Complexity – The joining of two or more systems, like the human body, family and various therapies.

8. Participation in care – The level at which the patient and family participate in all aspects of care.

Nurse Characteristics

In the Synergy Model, nursing care is a reflection of the integration of knowledge, skills, abilities and experience necessary to attend to the needs of patients and their families. As a result, nurse characteristics are derived from patient needs. They include:

1. Clinical judgment/clinical reasoning – AG-ACNPs should be skilled in making clinical decisions, ruling out differential diagnoses and thinking critically. They are also expected to have a broad grasp of the clinical scenario and must have the ability to combine both formal and informal knowledge with evidence-based guidelines.

2. Advocacy/moral agency – AG-ACNPs are expected to work on behalf of their patients, including the caregivers and nursing staff, and act as moral agents who can resolve clinical and ethical concerns both inside and outside the health-care setting.

3. Collaboration – AG-ACNPs must have the ability to function with others, like patients, health-care providers and families, with an attitude that encourages each person's contributions toward achieving optimal goals for the patient and family. Collaboration includes initiating referrals, providing consultation and coordinating intra- and interdisciplinary teams to develop patient-centered care plans.

4. Systems thinking – AG-ACNPs are expected to use clinical knowledge and skills that are useful in managing the available system and environmental resources in both health care and non-health-care settings. This knowledge is necessary to improve the patient's outcome by assessing and promoting cost-effective utilization of resources.

5. Response to diversity – AG-ACNPs are expected to recognize, use and appreciate the numerous differences in providing care for patients. These differences may include race, gender, ethnicity, spiritual beliefs, sexual orientation, age and socioeconomic status.

6. Facilitation of learning – AG-ACNPs are expected to promote formal and informal learning among patients and their families. They are also expected to promote learning among the nurses, other health-care workers and the community.

7. Clinical inquiry – AG-ACNPs must be involved in the process of providing evidence-based care. This includes evaluating practice and educating patients on the principles of care provided.

8. Caring practices – AG-ACNPs are expected to create a compassionate environment that is therapeutic for patients and supportive for staff. Caring practices do not only include engagement, responsiveness and engagement. They also include infection control, risk assessment, pain management and a healthy nurse/patient relationship.

Concepts of Caring

- Compassion – Compassion is an emotional capacity to share in someone's distress with a desire to alleviate it.
- Empathy – Empathy is the ability to stand in a speaker's shoes, see things from the speaker's perspective and communicate to the speaker that you understand his or her emotions.
- Sympathy – Sympathy is the ability to perceive another person's distress.
- Altruism – In the clinical setting, altruism is a voluntary and selfless action taken by a health worker to improve the welfare of a patient. These actions are usually not remunerated.

Sometimes, there may be no clear-cut line dividing all the concepts of care. An AG-ACNP can be both sympathetic and compassionate. In other cases, compassion can motivate an AG-ACNP to be altruistic, and vice versa.

Therapeutic Communication

In the nursing practice, therapeutic communication is a meaningful nurse/patient interaction that helps improve the patient's medical outcome. Therapeutic communication is an active process that requires effort and attention from both the speaker and the listener.

Therapeutic Communication Techniques

1. **Silence** – In this technique, the listener uses deliberate silence to give the speaker opportunity to express himself or herself. Deliberate silence eases tension, prevents conflicts, provides clarification and encourages self-expression.

2. **Accepting** – In this technique, the listener shows that s/he understands the speaker's emotions and affirms this to the speaker. The AG-ACNP may not agree with the patient but still acknowledges understanding.

3. **Offering self** – This technique is used for nonverbal communication. An AG-ACNP can offer time and attention to patients as a show of support. This can be as simple as keeping quiet to listen or staying behind after a shift to sit with a patient.

4. **Giving recognition** – In this technique, the listener acknowledges and draws attention to the actions of the speaker by pointing them out. This technique is useful for showing support and encouragement without using flattery or making judgments and evaluations.

5. **Giving broad openings** – This technique involves the use of open-ended questions. It allows the patient to lead the conversation and direct the flow and mood. An open question like "How are you today?" sets the pace for the patient.

6. **Making observations** – In this technique, the AG-ACNP notices the patient's demeanor, body language and facial expressions. This technique not only allows room for self-expression but helps the nurse notice any new symptoms.

7. **Placing the event in time or sequence** – In this technique, the AG-ACNP asks questions about the timing and occurrence of events. The aim is to get clarification and encourage the patient to recall more information.

8. **Focusing** – In this technique, the AG-ACNP focuses on important aspects of the patient's conversation and encourages him or her to talk about it.

9. **Reflecting** – An AG-ACNP uses this technique when a patient is seeking an evaluation or a solution to a problem. The nurse can direct the problem back to the patient by asking questions like "What do you think you should do?" This makes the patient responsible for his or her actions. It also improves self-awareness and reliance.

10. **Paraphrasing** – In this technique, the AG-ACNP interprets the emotional content of a patient's words and paraphrases the meaning back to show that what the patient said is understood. This technique encourages clarification and self-expression.

11. **Encouraging comparison** – In this technique, the AG-ACNP encourages the patient to recall similar experiences. The aim is to encourage the patient to think of solutions to challenges.

12. **Active listening** – This technique involves using prompts to engage and encourage the patient to go on talking. It shows that the AG-ACNP is paying attention. Examples of prompts include "Go on" and "I see."

13. **Seeking clarification** – The AG-ACNP uses this technique to clear up confusion or ambiguity. A statement like "I don't understand what you said" is a good example.

14. **Encouraging description of perception** – The AG-ACNP uses this technique with patients experiencing sensory hallucinations. This technique is non-judgmental and non-evaluative, and it gives patients freedom for self-expression.

15. **Voicing doubt** – This technique is used only after trust has been established. By expressing doubt, the AG-ACNP encourages the patient to take responsibility.

16. **Confronting** – This technique must only be used after trust is established. If used incorrectly, this technique can become a roadblock to effective communication. But when used correctly, it can help patients take responsibility.

17. **Restating** – This technique is used to show that the listener understands. In this technique, the AG-ACNP repeats the patient's exact words to show that the person was heard.

18. **Encouraging goal-setting** – The AG-ACNP uses this technique to encourage patients to be more involved and take responsibility. This technique requires tact because the nurse can unknowingly slip into evaluation and judgment.

19. **Encouraging the formulation of a plan of action** – This technique should only be used after trust is established. In this technique, the AG-ACNP encourages the patient to think of possible solutions to challenges.

20. **Limit-setting** – This technique should only be used after trust is established or when the patient shows inappropriate behavior. The AG-ACNP uses limit-setting to discourage inappropriate behavior and encourage appropriate behavior. For example, the nurse can say, "Please stop what you are doing. If you do not, I will leave."

21. **Suggesting collaboration** – In this technique, the AG-ACNP offers help to the patient. Offering unsolicited help can be a roadblock to therapeutic communication.

Distribution of Content in the Exam

1. Clinical Judgment (79%)
2. Advocacy/Moral Agency (3%)
3. Caring Practices (4%)
4. Response to Diversity (2%)
5. Facilitation of Learning (2%)
6. Collaboration (3%)
7. Systems Thinking (3%)
8. Clinical Inquiry (4%)

Clinical Judgment – This content makes up 79 percent of the test.

Core ACNP competencies

1. Creates new practice approaches that integrate research, theory and practice knowledge
2. Shows the highest level of accountability for professional practice
3. Practices independently, managing previously diagnosed and undiagnosed patients
4. Provides the full spectrum of health-care services, including health promotion, end-of-life care, disease prevention, palliative, health protection, counseling, anticipatory guidance and disease management
5. Uses advanced health assessment skills to differentiate normal findings from variations of normal and abnormal findings
6. Employs screening and diagnostic strategies in developing diagnoses

7. Prescribes medications within the scope of practice
8. Manages the health/illness status of patients and families over time.

AG-ACNP competencies

1. Uses theories, principles of practice and scientific information in differentiating between normal and abnormal changes in psychological, physiological and sociological functions and capacities
2. Functions as a licensed independent practitioner who can manage gerontology patients with critical, chronic and/or complex acute diseases, identify patients who are in emergent conditions and use physiological and technologic data to manage patients with abnormal and unstable physiological conditions and other life-threatening conditions
3. Provides health protection and encourages health promotion to patients by evaluating the risks present in patients with chronic, critical, acute or complex cases
4. Identifies comorbidities and patients at risk for physiological and mental deterioration, iatrogenesis and life-threatening conditions
5. Diagnoses common behavioral and mental health and substance use or addictive disorder/disease in the presence of complex acute, critical and chronic illness
6. Prioritizes diagnoses during rapid physiological and mental health deterioration or life-threatening instability
7. Performs specific diagnostic strategies and technical skills that monitor and sustain physiological function and ensure patient safety, including but not limited to X-ray interpretation, lumbar puncture, line and tube insertion, respiratory support, wound debridement and hemodynamic monitoring
8. Applies evidence-based practice in managing patients with unstable conditions and geriatric syndromes
9. Uses treatments and therapeutic devices when indicated, including oxygen, bilevel PAP, prosthetics, splints, Pacers, LVAD and other equipment
10. Performs therapeutic interventions that can stabilize acute and critical health problems, including but not limited to suturing, wound debridement, lumbar puncture, airway, line and tube insertion and management and others
11. Evaluates the effectiveness of speech therapy, palliative care, physical therapy, occupational therapy, home health, nutritional therapy and others
12. Implements interventions that can assist the patient with unstable and deteriorating clinical states and use the fundamentals of critical care support and advanced cardiac life support

13. Performs assessments on complex drug interactions, medical regimens, pharmacogenetic risks, adverse reactions and other forms of pharmacological assessment

14. Prescribes medications and monitors adverse drug outcomes and other medical dosages, particularly for vulnerable and high-risk patients

15. Uses pharmacological and non-pharmacological management strategies for behavioral and physical symptoms in individuals with psychiatric and substance abuse disorders

16. Practice within the scope of national licensing, including state licensing and institutional licensing (based on education, licensure and certification), and obeys the scope of practice for AG-ACNPs.

Patient Care Problems

A. Cardiovascular – This content makes up 17 percent of the test. Topics include:

1. **Acute coronary syndromes** – Heart conditions characterized by a sudden drop in blood flow to the heart include ST-elevation myocardial infarction, non-ST-elevation myocardial infarction and angina.
    A. STEMI – ST-elevation myocardial infarction (STEMI) is a serious form of a heart attack in which a major coronary vessel is completely blocked, and a portion of the heart does not receive blood supply.
    B. NSTEMI – A non-ST-elevation myocardial infarction is not as serious as a STEMI because the blockage of the coronary artery is temporal or partial.
    C. Percutaneous coronary intervention (PCI) – This used to be called angioplasty with stent. PCI is a non-operative procedure in which a catheter is passed through stenosed blood vessels to open them up.
    D. Thrombolytics – These are drugs used in treating patients with myocardial infarction to lyse blood clots. An example is a plasminogen activator (PA).

2. **Acute inflammatory disease** – Etiology, pathophysiology and pharmacology of acute inflammatory diseases of the heart.

3. **Cardiac surgery** – This includes:
    A. Revascularization – This is a surgical procedure that restores perfusion to an ischemic body part or organ. Examples are vascular bypass and angioplasty.
    B. Valve replacement – This is a surgical procedure for diseases and stenosed valves like the aortic valve, one of four valves that control blood flow through the heart.

C. Valve repair – The candidate will be assessed on knowledge of principles and complications of mitral, tricuspid and aortic valve repairs.

D. Hybrid procedures – The candidate is expected to know the principles of procedures that can be a mixture of surgical and interventional procedures.

E. Cardiopulmonary bypass pump – The candidate will be assessed on knowledge of the indications, principles and aftercare complications of the cardiopulmonary bypass pump.

4. **Cardiac arrest** – Principles of managing cardiac arrests, including ACLS protocol, the use of targeted temperature management, post-care, follow-up and others.

5. **Cardiac tamponade** – Pathophysiology, clinical features, acute management, follow-up and prognosis of cardiac tamponade.

6. **Cardiac trauma** – Different causes of blunt and penetrating trauma, their clinical features, acute management and follow-up.

7. **Cardiogenic shock** – Different causes of cardiogenic shock, its clinical presentation, investigations, resuscitative management and follow-up.

8. **Cardiomyopathies** – Etiology, pathogenesis, clinical features and management of hypertrophic, dilated, restrictive and idiopathic cardiomyopathy.

9. **Coronary artery disease** – Management of coronary artery disease caused by atherosclerosis.

10. **Dyslipidemia** – Different causes of dyslipidemia, including hyperlipidemia and liver diseases, as well as pathophysiology, clinical features and acute management.

11. **Dysrhythmia** – Types of dysrhythmias, pathophysiology and management.

12. **Heart failure** – Acute management of systolic, diastolic and congestive heart failure.

13. **Hypertension** – Pathophysiology and management of primary and secondary causes of hypertension.

14. **Hypertensive urgencies and emergencies** – Acute management of cerebrovascular diseases, pulmonary embolism, dissecting aortic aneurysm, myocardial infarction, heart failure, acute renal failure, hypertensive encephalopathy and others.

15. **Peripheral vascular insufficiency** – Pathophysiology and management of acute cases of arterial occlusion and carotid artery stenosis, as well as management options like endarterectomy, peripheral stents and femoral-popliteal bypass.

16. **Pulmonary edema** – Causes, pathophysiology and clinical presentation of pulmonary edema, emergency resuscitation methods, management and follow-up.

17. **Ruptured or dissecting aneurysm** – Pathophysiology, clinical features and management of ruptured and dissecting aneurysm.
18. **Structural heart defects** – Pathophysiology, clinical features and management of cyanotic and acyanotic congenital heart diseases
19. **Venous thromboembolism** – Causes of venous thromboembolism, risk factors for deep vein thrombosis, venous blood stasis and coagulation and acute management of venous thromboembolism.

B. Pulmonary – This content makes up 11 percent of the test. Topics include:

1. **Acute pulmonary embolus** – Deep vein thrombosis, venous coagulations and stasis; clinical features, like fast breathing, cyanosis, breathlessness, tachycardia and chest pain; and acute management, including oxygen therapy, thrombolytics and analgesia.
2. **Acute respiratory distress syndrome** – Different causes, pathophysiology, clinical features and treatment of acute respiratory distress syndrome.
3. **Acute respiratory failure** – Causes, pathophysiology, clinical features and treatment of acute respiratory failure.
4. **Air-leak syndromes** – Causes, pathophysiology, clinical features and treatment of pneumothorax, pneumopericardium and pneumomediastinum.
5. **Airway obstruction** – Pathophysiology, clinical features and treatment of angioedema, mucus plugs and airspace-occupying lesions.
6. **Aspirations** – Causes, pathophysiology and treatment for mucous, serous, bloody, purulent and serosanguinous pulmonary secretions.
7. **Asthma/restrictive airway disease** – Pathophysiology, clinical features and management of asthma, including status asthmaticus and other restrictive airway diseases, like bronchiolitis.
8. **Chronic lung diseases** – Pathophysiology, clinical features and management of chronic obstructive pulmonary diseases, like emphysema and chronic bronchitis.
9. **Obstructive sleep apnea** – Pathophysiology, clinical features and management of obstructive sleep apnea, including follow-up management.
10. **Pleural effusion** – Pathophysiology, clinical features and treatment of pleural effusion.
11. **Pulmonary arterial hypertension** – Pathophysiology, clinical features and treatment of pulmonary hypertension.
12. **Pulmonary infections** – Pathophysiology, clinical features and management of:
    A. Community-acquired pneumonia – Contracted outside the hospital. The most common causative pathogens are Streptococcus pneumonia,

Haemophilus influenza and atypical bacteria like legionella species, chlamydia pneumonia, viruses and mycoplasma pneumoniae.

B. Nosocomial pneumonia – Hospital-acquired pneumonia. Risk factors include immunosuppression, intubation, old age, immobility and sepsis. Nosocomial pneumonia is contracted by in-patients 48 to 72 hours after being admitted. It is generally caused by a bacterial infection rather than a virus. Implicated bacteria include rod-shaped gram-negative organisms like Pseudomonas aeruginosa, Klebsiella pneumoniae and Enterobacter spp; gram-positive bacteria, like Staphylococcus aureus; and Hemophilus influenzae. Implicated viruses include influenza, respiratory syncytial virus and cytomegalovirus.

C. Tuberculosis – Risk factors for pulmonary tuberculosis include immunosuppression as seen in cancer, chemotherapy and HIV. Tuberculosis is caused by mycobacterium spp.

D. Empyema – The collection of pus/abscessing in the lungs. Risk factors include pulmonary tuberculosis and other infectious suppurative lung diseases.

E. Ventilator-associated event – A new or progressive and persistent radiographic abnormality that develops in a patient on mechanical ventilation or within 48 hours of mechanical ventilation. The patient must also demonstrate one or more systemic signs, like fever, leukopenia, or leukocytosis, or have altered mental status if more than 70 years of age and have the following pulmonary criteria: dyspnea, rales, new-onset cough, increased respiratory secretions, impaired oxygenation and bronchial breath sounds.

F. Thoracic and pulmonary trauma and injuries – Lung contusions, hemothorax, fractured ribs and other blunt and penetrating injuries to the lungs.

13. **Thoracic surgery** – Principles, indications and complications of common thoracic surgeries, like lung reduction, pneumonectomy, lobectomy and others.

C. Endocrine Disorders – This content makes up 5 percent of the test. Topics include:

1. **Adrenal disorders** – This includes disorders of the adrenal cortex and medulla as seen in:

A. Cushing's disease – A disease of excess cortisol secretion. This overproduction can be caused by a tumor in the cortex of the adrenal gland that secretes excess cortisol. Apart from this, Cushing's disease can be caused by a tumor in the pituitary gland and ectopic tumors in the lungs, pancreas or thyroid gland.

    B. Addison's disease – An autoimmune disease of the adrenal glands that leads to insufficient secretion of cortisol and aldosterone.

    C. Congenital adrenal hyperplasia (CAH) – An adrenal disorder in which the body secretes too little cortisol. People with CAH can also have imbalances in aldosterone and androgen secretion. Their bodies might not make enough aldosterone but produce excess androgen.

    D. Hyperaldosteronism – A disorder of the adrenal gland characterized by excess aldosterone secretion. This hormone controls blood pressure and regulates the body's salt and potassium levels. Excess aldosterone is typically secreted by the adrenal glands or by tumors in the glands.

    E. Pheochromocytoma – A type of tumor found in the adrenal medulla, the inner part of the adrenal glands. This tumor secretes excess adrenaline. These tumors are typically noncancerous and do not spread to other sites in the body.

2. **Diabetes mellitus** – This includes knowledge of the pathophysiology, clinical features, diagnosis and management of:

    A. Type 1 diabetes – Characterized by autoimmune destruction of beta cells in the pancreas, total insulin deficiency, early age of onset and insulin dependence.

    B. Type 2 diabetes – Characterized by increasing insulin resistance, decreasing reception sensitivity to insulin, burnout of beta cells in the pancreas, obesity and varying levels of insulin dependence.

    C. Gestational diabetes – A disorder of glucose metabolism that develops with onset or first recognition during pregnancy. Most cases resolve with delivery.

    D. Others – These include genetic defects of beta cells, genetic defects in insulin action, diseases of the exocrine pancreas, endocrinopathies, infections and genetic syndromes associated with diabetes.

3. **Diabetic ketoacidosis (DKA)/hyperglycemic hyperosmolar state (HHS)**

    A. Diabetic ketoacidosis – This is an endocrine emergency characterized by metabolic acidosis, hyperglycemia, ketonemia and severe dehydration. It is a common complication of type 1 diabetes mellitus.

    B. Hyperglycemic hyperosmolar state – Hyperosmolar hyperglycemic state (HHS) is an acute complication of diabetes mellitus characterized by hyperglycemia, hyperosmolarity, dehydration and ketoacidosis. Symptoms include dehydration, altered sensorium, weakness, visual disturbances and leg cramps.

4. **<u>Hyperglycemia</u>** – This condition involves high blood sugar that is measured as 180 mg/dL two hours after eating or a fasting blood sugar that is greater than 125 mg/dL. It is a common feature of diabetes mellitus.

5. **<u>Hypoglycemia</u>** – This condition involves blood sugar that is less than 70 mg/dL.

6. **<u>Syndrome of inappropriate secretion of antidiuretic hormone (SIADH)</u>** – SIADH is an excess secretion of the antidiuretic hormone (ADH) from the pituitary gland and other nonpituitary sources and its excessive stimulation of vasopressin receptors. As a result, there is an impaired excretion of water and consequent hyponatremia and hypervolemia. Causes include nephrogenic SIADH; disturbances of the central nervous system, like stroke; hemorrhage; trauma; infection; mental disorders, including psychosis; cancers; and medications that can stimulate the release or effect of ADH. These implicated drugs include selective serotonin reuptake inhibitors, cyclophosphamide, chlorpropamide, oxcarbazepine and carbamazepine. The action of carbamazepine and oxcarbazepine includes increasing the sensitivity of renal tubule receptors to ADH.

7. **<u>Thyroid disorders</u>** – Thyroid disorders include hyperthyroidism and hypothyroidism.
   A. Hyperthyroidism – Excess secretion of thyroid hormone. Features include toxic goiter, weight loss, heat intolerance, tremors, oculopathies, palpitations, infertility, alopecia and diarrhea.
   B. Hypothyroidism – Insufficient secretion of thyroid hormone. Features include goiter, weight gain, fatigue, infertility, cold intolerance and others.

D. Hematology/Immunology/Oncology – This content makes up 5 percent
of the test. Topics include:

1. **<u>Anemia</u>** – Pathophysiology, clinical features and management of different classes of anemia, such as:
   A. Microcytic anemia – Most iron deficiency anemias as seen in malnutrition, chronic kidney disease, chronic blood loss, pregnancy, parasitic worm infestations, chronic diseases, malignancies, malabsorption syndromes and others.
   B. Macrocytic anemia – As seen in megaloblastic anemia caused by a deficiency or an impaired utilization of vitamin B12 or B9; and in non-megaloblastic anemia, as seen in liver diseases, hypothyroidism, alcoholism and myelodysplastic syndrome.

2. **Anticoagulation** – Principles and practice of anticoagulation therapies for patients with clotting disorders and coagulopathies. Also, assessment of the indications, contraindications and complications, side effects and adverse effects of anticoagulation therapies.
3. **Autoimmune diseases** – Lupus, antiphospholipid antibody syndrome, vasculitis and polyarteritis nodosa.
4. **Blood and blood-product administration** – Principles and practice of blood and blood component transfusion. Some of these include indications, monitoring, correction, incompatibilities, correction and complications.

Blood components
   A. Plasma – Plasma is the fluid component of blood in which all the blood cells are suspended. Plasma makes up 55 percent of the total blood volume. About 90 percent of plasma is composed of water, which acts as a solvent for salts, lipids, hormones, immunoglobulins, clotting factors, fibrinogen and albumin. Plasma is used to transport blood cells, water and nutrients; maintain the body's homeostasis; provide a natural defense against infections and aid in blood coagulation. Albumin is used to maintain oncotic pressure in the intravascular space. Albumin also transports blood components and nutrients. Immunoglobulins mount responses to various infectious pathogens, and clotting factors present in plasma help stimulate hemostasis and blood coagulation. Serum has the same constituents as plasma except for clotting factors and fibrinogen.
   B. Red blood cells – Red blood cells make up about 37 to 43 percent of blood volume. Red blood cells are the oxygen-carrying component of the blood. A drop of blood contains approximately five million red blood cells. Red blood cells are small anucleated biconcave disks that carry hemoglobin. Hemoglobin gives red blood cells their characteristic red color.
   C. Platelets – Platelets/thrombocytes make up less than 1 percent of the total blood volume and are smaller in size than white blood cells and red blood cells. Platelets are involved in the coagulation and hemostasis of the blood. When a blood vessel ruptures, the platelets combine with fibrin to form platelet plugs.
   D. White blood cells – White blood cells make up less than 1 percent of the total blood volume. There are about 6,000 to 8,000 white blood cells per cubic milliliter of blood. White blood cells are slightly larger than red blood cells and are important aspects of the immune system.

Use of blood products/components
   A. Packed red blood cells – Red blood cells are used for acute hemorrhage, hemorrhagic shock and severe anemia. A unit of packed red blood cells is

expected to increase a patient's hematocrit by 3 percent. Packed red blood cells are obtained from centrifuged whole blood.

B. Fresh-frozen plasma – Fresh-frozen plasma is given to patients with clotting disorders caused by insufficient or defective clotting factors. Fresh-frozen plasma is also administered to patients with low INR, such as patients on warfarin/heparin therapy.

C. Cryoprecipitate – Cryoprecipitate is obtained from plasma and contains fibrinogen, Factor VIII, Factor XII, Von Willebrand Factor and fibronectin. This blood product is used for patients with insufficient fibrinogen levels. It is also used for hemophiliacs.

D. Platelets – Platelets are given to patients with severe thrombocytopenia, such as those who have aplastic anemia.

E. Albumin – Albumin is given to increase the oncotic pressure of blood. Oncotic pressure prevents the permeability of blood vessels and tissue edema. Albumin is useful in patients in hypovolemic shock, as seen in severe burns. Albumin is also useful for patients with pre-renal acute renal failure.

Complications of blood transfusion

1. Acute complications of blood transfusion – Acute complications occur within 24 hours of a blood transfusion. They include acute hemolytic reaction, anaphylactic reaction, coagulopathies caused by massive transfusion, febrile non-hemolytic reaction, transfusion-associated circulatory overload, urticarial reaction, transfusion-related acute lung injury and sepsis.

2. Delayed complications of blood transfusion – These transfusion reactions occur more than 24 hours after a blood transfusion. This can take days, months and even years. Examples are delayed hemolytic reaction, post-transfusion purpura, iron overload, microchimerism, overtransfusion and transfusion-related immunomodulation.

5. **<u>Coagulopathies</u>** – Pathophysiology, clinical features and management of coagulopathies, like thrombocytopenia DIC and hypercoagulable states as seen in the use of female hormones like estrogens and birth control pills; a postoperative period of the hip, knee and genitourinary surgeries; pregnancy; phospholipid antibodies in blood cancer; elevated homocysteine levels; and protein deficiencies of factor V Leiden, antithrombin III, protein S, protein C and others.

6. **<u>Hematologic and solid tumors</u>** – Pathophysiology, clinical features, diagnosis and treatment of hematologic malignancies like leukemia, multiple myeloma, aplastic anemia and solid organ tumors.

7. **Immunosuppression** – Pathophysiology, clinical features and management of immunosuppression caused by organ transplantation, cancers, chemotherapeutic drugs and others.
8. **Myelosuppression** – Bone marrow suppression as seen in neutropenia, pancytopenia and thrombocytopenia.

E. Gastrointestinal – This makes up 5 percent of the test. Topics include:

1. **Abdominal trauma** – Pathophysiology, clinical features and acute management of blunt and penetrating abdominal injuries.
2. **Bowel infarction/obstruction/perforation** –Etiology, pathophysiology, clinical features and management of bowel infarction, obstruction and perforation.
3. **Gallbladder disease** – Gall bladder stones, carcinoma of the gall bladder, cholecystitis, choledocholithiasis, biliary dyskinesia, sclerosing cholangitis, gallbladder polyps and others.
4. **Gastroesophageal reflux** – Etiology, pathophysiology, clinical features and management of gastroesophageal reflux.
5. **GI infectious disorders**
   A. Bacterial – Salmonella, shigella, H. Pylori, Campylobacter, E.coli, Vibrio cholera, Clostridium difficile.
   B. Viral – Adenoviruses, rotavirus, norovirus, Hepatitis A and E viruses.
   C. Parasitic – Worm infestations such as hookworm, tapeworm, roundworm, pinworm infestations, amoebiasis, schistosomiasis and others.
6. **GI hemorrhage** – Upper GI hemorrhage as seen in gastritis, peptic ulcer disease, Mallory Weiss tears and ruptured esophageal varices. Lower GI hemorrhage as seen in hemorrhoids, rectal tears, intestinal cancers, inflammatory bowel disease and others.
7. **GI motility disorders** – Constipation, diarrhea, ileus and gastroparesis.
8. **GI surgeries** – Principles and practice, including contraindications, indications, complications and risk factors of surgeries like laparoscopies, laparotomies, colectomies, appendectomies, gastrectomies and others.
9. **Hepatorenal syndrome** – Type 1 hepatorenal syndrome (HRS) characterized by rapidly deteriorating kidney failure as evidenced by a doubling of serum creatinine to levels greater than 221 µmol/L, or a halving of the creatinine clearance to less than 20 mL/min over less than two weeks. Prognosis is poor, with mortality rates greater than 50 percent after one month.
Type 2 HRS has a slow onset and is not associated with an inciting event. There is an increased serum creatinine level to more than 133 µmol/L or a creatinine clearance of less than 40 mL/min and urine sodium < 10 µmol/L. It also has a

poor outlook, with a median survival of approximately six months if there is no liver transplantation.

10. **Liver disease** – Infectious liver diseases (e.g., hepatitis A, B, C, D and E), alcoholic fatty liver disease, nonalcoholic fatty liver disease, infiltrative diseases (e.g., Wilson's disease), hemochromatosis, amyloidosis, sarcoidosis, liver carcinomas, disorders of the biliary tract and hepatic vasculature and others.

11. **Nausea/vomiting** – Etiology, pathophysiology and management of nausea and vomiting.

12. **Nutrition** – Causes, pathophysiology, clinical features and treatment of both macro and micro malnutrition, as well as principles and practice of enteral and parenteral nutrition.

13. **Pancreatitis** – Caused by gallstones, heavy alcohol consumption, blunt and penetrating trauma, mumps, tumors, cystic fibrosis, hypertriglyceridemia, hypercalcemia, smoking, infections and medications. Diagnosis of acute pancreatitis is by a threefold increase in serum amylase or lipase. These tests may be normal in chronic pancreatitis.

14. **Peptic ulcer disease** – Pathophysiology, clinical features and management of gastric and duodenal ulcers.

F. Renal/Genitourinary – This makes up 6 percent of the test. Topics include:

1. **Acute kidney failure** – Parameters include an increase in sCr ≥0.3 mg/dL (≥26.5 μmol/L) within 48 hours; or an increase in sCr ≥1.5 times baseline, which is confirmed or suspected to have occurred within the prior seven days; or urine volume <0.5 mL/kg/h for six hours.

   A. Renal causes – Acute glomerulonephritis, nephrotic syndrome, pyelonephritis, interstitial tubular necrosis, diabetic, hypertensive, HIV-induced nephropathy, renal carcinoma, infiltrative diseases and others.

   B. Prerenal causes – Cardiogenic shock, hypovolemic shock, acute hemorrhage, severe dehydration, burns, anaphylactic shock, sepsis, poisoning and others.

   C. Post renal causes – Obstructive uropathy caused by renal stones, posterior urethra valves, urethral strictures, benign prostatic hyperplasia, prostate carcinoma, bladder carcinoma and others.

2. **Chronic kidney disease** (CKD) – The five stages of kidney disease are:
   A. Stage 1 – Normal or high GFR > 90 mL/min
   B. Stage 2 – Mild CKD in which GFR is 60–89 mL/min
   C. Stage 3A – Moderate CKD in which GFR is 45–59 mL/min
   D. Stage 3B – Moderate CKD in which GFR is 30–44 mL/min

E. Stage 4 – Severe CKD in which GFR is 15–29 mL/min

F. Stage 5 – End-stage CKD in which GFR is <15 mL/min

3. **Contrast-associated nephropathy** – This occurs when serum creatinine (Scr) is raised to more than 25 percent or ≥0.5 mg/dl (44 μmol/l) from the normal in 48 hours. Risk factors include diabetes mellitus and underlying chronic kidney disease (e.g., estimated glomerular filtration rate (eGFR) <60 ml/min), age > 75 years, uncontrolled hypertension, congestive heart failure, liver cirrhosis, hypoalbuminemia and use of intra-aortic balloon pump. Procedure-related factors, like repeated exposures to CM within 72 hours, high-contrast volume, osmolality and viscosity of the contrast. Other factors that can increase the risk include the concomitant use of diuretics or nephrotoxic drugs, such as NSAIDs and aminoglycosides.

4. **Fluid and electrolyte imbalances** – These include:
   A. Hyperkalemia – Acute kidney injury, chronic kidney injury, use of potassium-sparing diuretics, rhabdomyolysis, burns, hemolysis and others.
   B. Hypokalemia – Gastroenteritis, laxative abuse, malabsorption, fistula, colostomy, hyperglycemia, hyperaldosteronism, renal tubular acidosis, metabolic alkalosis, total parenteral nutrition, dialysis, plasmapheresis and others.
   C. Hypernatremia – Dehydration, iatrogenic causes, excessive sodium intake, Cushing syndrome, hyperaldosteronism, peritoneal dialysis, vomiting, diarrhea, fistula, diabetes insipidus, osmotic diuresis as seen in alcohol intoxication, burns and others.
   D. Hyponatremia – Chronic kidney diseases, cirrhosis, heart failure, diuretic therapy, mineralocorticoid deficiency, SIADH, burns, pancreatitis and others.
   E. Hypercalcemia – Primary hyperparathyroidism, multiple myeloma, exogenous vitamin D, bedridden patients, thyrotoxicosis, Paget's disease, vitamin A toxicity, adrenal insufficiency and others.
   F. Hypocalcemia – Vitamin D insufficiency, hypoparathyroidism, malabsorption syndromes, insufficient calcium intake and others.
   G. Dehydration – Mild, moderate and severe dehydration causes include metabolic acidosis, hypernatremia, gastroenteritis, hyperpyrexia, burns, heatstroke and others.
   H. Edema – Congestive heart failure, liver failure, kidney diseases, nephrotic syndrome and others.

5. **Infections** – Complicated and uncomplicated upper and lower urinary tract infections, pelvic inflammatory diseases and sexually transmitted infections.

G. Integumentary – This makes up 2 percent of the test. Topics include:

1. **Exfoliative skin disorders** – These include:
   A. Stevens-Johnson (SJS) – Etiology, pathophysiology, clinical features and management of patients with SJS.
   B. Toxic epidermal necrolysis (TEN) – Etiology, pathophysiology, clinical features and management of patients with TEN.
   C. Stevens-Johnson/TEN – Etiology, pathophysiology, clinical features and management of patients with SJS/TEN.

2. **Infectious skin disorders** – These include:
   A. Necrotizing fasciitis – Caused by group A streptococcus. Others include Aeromonas hydrophila, clostridium, E. coli, Klebsiella and staphylococcus aureus.
   B. Cellulitis – Caused commonly by staphylococcus aureus and streptococcus.

3. **Intravenous infiltration and extravasation** – These are complications of intravenous therapy. Infiltration occurs when a non-vesicant IV fluid or medications leak into the surrounding tissue. Causes are improper placement or dislodgement of the catheter. Extravasation occurs when a vesicant drug leaks into the surrounding tissue. Extravasation can be severe and can cause tissue necrosis and loss of function in an extremity.

4. **Pressure ulcers/pressure injuries** – Risks include pressure, friction and shearing. Risk factors include immobility, incontinence, lack of sensory perception, poor nutrition and impaired blood flow.

5. **Wounds** – Classification of wounds
   A. Class 1 wounds – These are clean and uninfected wounds that have no inflammation and are primarily closed. These wounds do not invade the respiratory, genital, alimentary or urinary tracts. Closed drains are used for draining fluid.
   B. Class 2 wounds – These are both contimnated wounds and clean wounds without contamination. However, they penetrate the urinary, respiratory, gastrointestinal and genital tracts under controlled situations, such as surgery.

C. Class 3 wounds – These are contaminated wounds that are fresh and open either from a disruption to sterile surgical techniques or seepage from the alimentary tract into the wound.

D. Class 4 wounds – These are dirty and infected wounds caused by improper care. These wounds contain dead and necrotic tissue and are typically caused by the action of microorganisms on perforated viscera or during surgery.

H. Musculoskeletal – This makes up 4 percent of the test. Topics include:

1. **Neuromuscular dysfunction related to illness** – Examples are diabetic neuropathy; motor neuron diseases like amyotrophic lateral sclerosis; toxic neuropathy; small fiber neuropathy; autonomic neuropathies; hereditary muscular disorders, like congenital myopathies; muscular dystrophy; metabolic myopathies; acquired muscular disorders like inclusion body myositis; dermatomyositis; polymyositis; necrotizing myopathy; neuromuscular junction disorders like myasthenia gravis; and Lambert-Eaton Syndrome.

2. **Mobility** – This includes disorders that cause immobility, debility and falls. Examples are:
    A. Arthritis – Inflammation of the joints. Types include rheumatoid arthritis, osteoarthritis, septic arthritis, psoriatic arthritis and autoimmune diseases.
    B. Amputation – Surgical removal of a limb or part of a limb. The most common indication is gangrene. Other indications include cancerous tumors of the limb, fulminant infection of the limb, diabetic foot ulcers, frostbite, pneumococcal meningitis, neuromas and others.
    C. Birth defects – Limb reduction refers to congenital birth defects of the upper and lower limbs. In this case, the affected limbs fail to grow properly due to factors like impaired blood flow to the affected area. Risk factors include cord band syndrome, radiation exposure, tobacco and alcohol use during pregnancy and exposure to viruses and chemicals.
    D. Cerebral palsy – An irreversible and non-progressive disorder of motor function caused by an injury to a developing brain. Risk factors include birth asphyxia, kernicterus, exposure of the fetus to any TORCHES infection, neonatal hypoglycemia, exposure of the fetus to heavy metals and chemicals, meningitis and head injuries.
    E. Spinal cord injury – Paralysis is the total or complete loss of spinal cord function. Examples include paraplegia, which is a loss of sensory and motor function in the lower limbs. This condition occurs when an injury is from the thoracic spine and below. Quadriplegia is a complete loss of

function in the upper and lower limbs due to injury at the cervical spine, C1–C8.

F. Multiple sclerosis – An autoimmune disease of the central nervous system that leads to demyelination of nerve fibers.

3. **Gait disturbances** – Gait disturbances include:
   A. Hemiplegic gait – This is commonly seen in patients with stroke. The patient presents with flexion, internal rotation and adduction of the affected arm. The ipsilateral leg is extended, and the toes and foot are plantar-flexed. On walking, the patient holds the arm to a side and drags the affected leg in circumduction.
   B. Diplegic gait – This is seen in patients with cerebral palsy. There is space in both the upper and lower limbs, and the patient presents by dragging both legs and scraping the toes.
   C. Neuropathic gait – Also called equine gait or steppage gait, it occurs in a patient with foot drop. The patient tries to raise the affected leg as high as possible to avoid dragging it on the floor. Unilateral causes include amyotrophic lateral sclerosis, peripheral neuropathies, Charcot-Marie-Tooth disease and others.
   D. Myopathic gait – This gait is seen in patients with myopathies like muscular dystrophy. Weakness in the muscles of the hip girdle causes the pelvis on the contralateral side to drop. This is called the Trendelenburg sign. If there is bilateral weakness on both hip joints, the hips droop when walking, causing a waddling gait.
   E. Choreiform gait – This is called hyperkinetic gait. This is seen in patients with basal ganglia disorders like Sydenham's chorea, athetosis, Huntington's disease, chorea and dystonia. Affected patients develop irregular, jerky and involuntary movements in the upper and lower limbs.
   F. Ataxic gait (cerebella gait) – This is seen in disorders affecting the cerebellum. Patients display a clumsy and staggering movement that has a wide-based stance. The patient may also demonstrate titubation, staggering back and forth and from side to side when standing.
   G. Parkinsonian gait – The patient presents with rigidity and bradykinesia. The patient also stoops with the head and neck forward and flexes at the knees. The patient demonstrates *marche a petit pas.*
   H. Sensory gait – Patients with this gait have impaired proprioception and slam their foot hard on the ground to have a sense of its position. This gait is typically called stomping gait and is seen in patients with diabetic neuropathy, vitamin B12 deficiency and tabes dorsalis.

4. **Infections** – Etiology, pathophysiology, clinical features and management of infectious diseases, like necrotizing fasciitis and osteomyelitis.
5. **Rhabdomyolysis** – Etiology, pathophysiology, clinical features and management of rhabdomyolysis.
6. **Traumatic fractures** – Etiology, pathophysiology, clinical features and management of the different types of open and closed fractures.

I. Neurology – This makes up 7 percent of the test. Topics include:

1. **Encephalopathy** – Etiology, pathophysiology, clinical features and management of encephalopathy. Common causes include malignant hypertension, uremia, hepatic encephalopathy, sepsis, heavy metal poisoning, electrolyte imbalance, alcohol intoxication, metabolic disorders and others.
2. **Head trauma** – Etiology, pathophysiology, clinical features and management of blunt and penetrating head trauma
3. **Herniation syndromes** – These include:
    A. Transtentorial herniation – Also called uncal herniation, it involves a unilateral mass squeezing the temporal lobe over and under the tentorium.
    B. Subfalcine herniation – An expanding mass in the cerebral hemisphere pushes the cingulate gyrus under the falx cerebelli.
    C. Central herniation – Bilateral mass effects cause both temporal lobes to herniate through the tentorial notch.
    D. Upward transtentorial herniation – An infratentorial mass pushes on the brain stem and causes brain stem ischemia.
    E. Tonsillar herniation – An expanding mass in the infratentorial pushes the cerebellar tonsils through the foramen magnum.

4. **Intracerebral hemorrhage/intraventricular hemorrhage** – Causes include hypertension, arteriovenous malformation, cocaine use, penetrating head trauma, tumors, sarcoidosis and others.
5. **Intracranial hypertension** – Causes include idiopathic intracranial hypertension, chronic subdural hematoma, brain tumors, meningoencephalitis, hydrocephalus arteriovenous malformation, venous sinus thrombosis and others.
6. **Neurologic infectious diseases** – These diseases include meningitis, encephalitis and meningoencephalitis.
7. **Neuromuscular disorders** – Management of disorders affecting the neuromuscular junctions.
8. **Seizure disorders** – Etiology, pathophysiology and management of seizure disorders.

9. **Space-occupying lesions** – Pathophysiology, clinical features and management of space-occupied lesions, like tumors, intracerebral hemorrhage, edema, pus and others.
10. **Spinal cord injury** – Etiology and pathophysiology of spinal cord injuries.
11. **Stroke** – Pathophysiology and management of both ischemic and hemorrhagic strokes.
12. **Traumatic brain injury** – Includes both blunt and traumatic injury to the brain.

J. Psychosocial/Behavioral/Cognitive Health – This makes up 4 percent of the test. Topics include:

1. Agitation – Making a diagnosis of agitation, collecting a detailed clinical history to rule out the likely cause of agitation, requesting the necessary diagnostic investigations and commencing treatment. In some cases, the use of physical or chemical restraints is necessary to reduce self-harm and/or assault on the staff.

2. Anxiety disorders
   A. Generalized anxiety disorder – Patients have excessive worry or anxiety that lasts for a minimum of six months. Sources of anxiety are health, social interactions, work and other life activities. Symptoms include restlessness, agitation, easy fatigability, lack of concentration, insomnia, muscle tension and others.
   B. Panic disorder – Affected individuals have recurrent and unexpected sudden episodes of panic attacks and unexpected episodes of intense fear that build up quickly. Attacks can be expected or caused by certain triggers. Symptoms include palpitations, sweating, shaking, difficulty in breathing/fast breathing, hyperventilation, a feeling of doom or a feeling of things getting out of control.
   C. Phobia-related disorders – A phobia is an intense fear of specific situations or/and objects. In phobias, the level of fear is out of proportion to the danger caused by the object/situation. Symptoms include excessive worry, anxiety, panic or a feeling of impending doom. There are different types of phobias, some of which are fear of heights, spiders, blood, flying and others.
   D. Social anxiety disorder – This is also known as social phobia. Affected individuals have a deep fear of social situations. They worry that their actions may be negatively interpreted by others. This leads to embarrassment, worry and avoidance of social gatherings.
   E. Separation anxiety disorder – Affected individuals are afraid of being separated from people they are attached to. This is often seen in young children, but it can also be seen in adults. Affected individuals may experience nightmares about separation from their attachment figures. They may also experience physical symptoms when separated or when anticipating a separation.

F. Selective mutism – This is a rare anxiety disorder in which people are unable to speak in certain social situations. Affected individuals have normal language skills. Selective mutism usually occurs in children who are less than five years. It is also associated with extreme shyness, clinging behavior, compulsive traits and temper tantrums.

3. Delirium – This consists of acute, short-lived and typically reversible fluctuations in attention, cognition and consciousness level.

A. The causes of delirium include drugs, such as anticholinergics, psychoactive drugs and opioids; dehydration; CNS infections and tumors; vitamin deficiencies; withdrawal symptoms; and vascular, metabolic, hematologic and endocrinologic disorders.
B. Factors that put an individual at risk for delirium include brain pathologies like dementia, stroke and Parkinson's. Other factors are old age, alcohol intoxication and sensory impairment of vision and/or hearing.
C. The following can trigger delirium in at-risk groups: infection, dehydration, shock, anemia, hypoxia, immobility, malnutrition, use of urinary catheters, pain, sleep deprivation and stress, hepatic encephalopathy, renal encephalopathy and recent exposure to anesthetic drugs.

4. Dementia – This is a chronic, widespread and usually irreversible deterioration of cognition. Classification of dementia includes:

A. Alzheimer's or non-Alzheimer type, irreversible and reversible, cortical or subcortical and common or rare.
B. The types of dementia include Alzheimer's disease, HIV-associated dementia, dementia with Lewy bodies, vascular dementia and frontotemporal dementia. It is also seen in patients with Huntington's disease, Parkinson's disease, Creutzfeldt-Jakob disease, metabolic diseases, prion disorders, subdural hematomas, normal pressure hydrocephalus, progressive supranuclear palsy, neurosyphilis, brain tumors located in the cognitive parts of the subcortical and cortical regions, Gerstmann-Sträussler-Scheinker syndrome, chronic traumatic encephalopathy and poisonings with heavy metals.

5. Maltreatment – Maltreatment is common among dependents like children and the elderly. Examples of maltreatment include:

A. Abuse – Can be physical, emotional, sexual or medical (Munchausen by proxy).
B. Neglect – The failure to meet the basic physical, emotional, educational and medical needs of a dependent.

C. Self-harm – An intentional injury of one's own body, without the intention of causing suicide. Risk factors for self-harm include substance abuse, psychotic illness, bipolar disorder, anxiety disorder and others.

6. Medication nonadherence – The failure to take a prescription drug correctly, according to the dosage, timing and duration. Causes of medication non-adherence include the inability to pay for drugs, chronicity of the disease, poor health education, polypharmacy, side effects of the drugs, functional impairments, cognitive impairments and mental illness.

7. Mood disorders – These include:

A. Bipolar disorder – This disorder involves alternating episodes of mania and depression. However, patients may have a predominance of one or the other. Classification of bipolar disorders includes bipolar I disorder, which is defined by the presence of at least one full-fledged manic episode and usually depressive episodes; bipolar II disorder, which is defined by major depressive episodes with at least one hypomanic episode and no full-fledged manic episodes; and unspecified bipolar disorder, which has clear bipolar features that do not meet the specific criteria for other bipolar disorders.

B. Depression – These disorders are characterized by severe and persistent sadness that interferes with function. Classification of depression includes major depressive disorder, which is a persistent depressive disorder that lasts for more than two years even with medication; other specified or unspecified depressive disorder; and classification by etiology, which includes premenstrual dysphoric disorders; depressive disorder due to another medical condition and substance/medication-induced depressive disorder.

8. Post-ICU syndrome – Post-intensive care syndrome is a group of physical, mental and emotional symptoms that persist in a patient who has left the intensive care unit.

Cognitive symptoms include difficulty talking, decreased memory, memory loss, poor concentration and sleep disorders. These symptoms may last for weeks, months and even years after discharge from the ICU.

9. Sleep disorders – These include insomnia, parasomnia, idiopathic hypersomnia and sleep disorders involving the circadian rhythm.

A. Insomnia – Difficulty falling or staying asleep, early awakening or having a sensation of unrefreshing sleep.

B. Excessive daytime sleepiness – The tendency to fall asleep during normal waking hours.

C. Narcolepsy – A sleep disorder characterized by chronic, excessive daytime sleepiness, with associated cataplexy, sleep paralysis and hypnagogic and hypnopompic hallucinations.
D. Parasomnia – Undesirable behaviors that occur as a person is about to sleep, is sleeping or is aroused from sleep. They include somnambulism, sleep terrors, nightmares, REM sleep disorders and sleep-related leg cramps.
E. Idiopathic hypersomnia – Excessive daytime sleepiness with or without a long sleep time. There is no narcolepsy, cataplexy, hypnagogic hallucinations or sleep paralysis.
F. Circadian rhythm sleep disorders – Sleep disorders that are caused by desynchronization between the internal sleep-wake rhythms and the light-darkness cycle. Affected individuals have insomnia or excessive daytime sleepiness, or both. All these resolve as the body clock realigns itself. Examples include jet lag, shift work disorder and altered sleep phase types.

10. Substance abuse – This is a spectrum of substance-related disorders in which the affected individuals persist in using a substance despite experiencing significant problems associated with its use. These problems can be physical, mental or psychological.

The likelihood for a drug to become addictive is dependent on:

A. The route of its administration
B. The rate at which it passes the blood-brain barrier
C. The rate at which it stimulates the reward pathway
D. The time of onset
E. Its ability to create tolerance or withdrawal symptoms.

11. Suicidal behavior – This includes completed suicide and attempted suicide.

A. Completed suicide – This is a suicidal act that results in death.
B. Attempted suicide – This is a nonfatal but injurious act that is self-directed and intended to result in death. It may or may not cause injury.
C. Nonsuicidal self-injury (NSSI) – This is a self-inflicted injurious act that is not intended to cause death. The causes of suicidal behavior include depression; other mental disorders, like schizophrenia and bipolar disorder; alcohol and substance abuse; previous suicide attempts; unemployment and economic repression; personality disorders; impulsivity; traumatic childhood experiences; family history of suicide and/mental disorders and others.

K. Factors Influencing Health Status – This makes up 3 percent of the test.
Topics include:

1. **Advance care planning** – In advance care planning, patients are allowed to make decisions about their health-care management plans in the case of crises. These decisions are often based on the patient's values and discussions with loved ones and caregivers.

   The principles of advance care planning include education on the life-sustaining treatments available, making decisions on the forms of preferential treatment in the event of a life-limiting illness, discussing such plans with loved ones and caregivers and filling out the advance directives forms.

   An advance directive is a written statement of a patient's preferential medical treatment at the end of life. It includes a living will, which is a legal document that states the forms of treatment a patient prefers if they are no longer able to give consent. These treatment options include resuscitation and other end-of-life-treatment. A health-care proxy or durable power of attorney for health care is a document that states the patient's appointed attorney in cases when the patient is unable to give consent. A durable power of attorney does not nullify the living will. Medical orders for life-sustaining treatment (MOLST) or provider orders for life-sustaining treatment (POLST) are documents that contain the patient's medical orders for end-of-life treatment.

2. **Cancer prevention and screening** – Examples of cancer screening include:
   A. Cervical cancer screening – Screening tests for the prevention and early detection of cervical cancer are the Pap test and the HPV test. The Pap test is done to check for precancerous changes in the cervix. These precancerous changes can transform into cervical cancer if they are not treated early. The HPV test is done to assess for the cancerous strains of the human papillomavirus, which are HPV 16 and 18.
   B. Breast cancer screening – Screening for breast cancer includes breast self-examination, breast mammography and breast MRI.
   C. Prostate cancer screening – Prostate cancer is a common cause of cancer in middle-aged men. Although there are no definite screening methods for prostate cancer, the two methods are the prostate-specific antigen and digital rectal examination. Prostate-specific antigen measures the level of PSA in the blood. PSA levels can be higher in men with cancer. However, it can also be elevated in other non-cancerous causes, like infections, use of certain medications, some procedures and other non-cancerous causes of prostate enlargement. Digital rectal examination (DRE) is the examination of the prostate via the anus. For the examination, a clinician inserts a gloved and well-lubricated finger into the anus to examine features of the prostate, such as its size, consistency, texture and attachment to surrounding structures.

D. Colorectal cancer screening – Colorectal cancer is cancer of the colon and/or rectum. Screening options for colorectal cancer include stool tests (fecal occult blood test, fecal immunochemical test and stool DNA test), flexible sigmoidoscopy, colonoscopy and CT colonography.

Screening is necessary for these at-risk groups: family history of colorectal polyps or colorectal cancer; history of Crohn's disease and other inflammatory bowel diseases; history of syndromes like familial adenomatous polyposis.

Some prevention principles include the reduction of risk factors like tobacco, alcohol, environmental pollution, occupational carcinogens, radiation, sedentary lifestyle, infections and others.

3. **Caregiver burden** – This is used to describe the physical, mental, psychological and financial stress a caregiver experiences in providing care for a sick loved one. In providing care for gerontology patients, the AG-ACNP is expected to identify the features of stress among caregivers and help in its management. Some features of caregiver burden include:
   A. Feeling overwhelmed, worried, fatigued,
   B. Suffering from insomnia, irritability and emotional outbursts
   C. Depression, anxiety
   D. Frequent headaches, body pains
   E. Weight loss, weight gain.

Management options for affected individuals include counseling, support groups, social support, relaxation techniques and medications.

4. **Comorbid risk reduction** – This involves system-specific screening. Examples include:
   A. Tumor markers – These are biomarkers that are found in blood, urine or body tissues and whose concentrations are raised by the presence of one or more types of cancer. Tumor markers can be realized by the cancerous cells or by surrounding tissues as a response to the tumor. Examples of tumor markers include alpha-fetoprotein, which is used to screen for germ cell tumors and hepatocellular carcinoma; CA15-3 and CA 27-29, which are used to screen for breast cancer; human chorionic gonadotropin, which is used to screen for choriocarcinoma and other gestational trophoblastic diseases; and others.
   B. Enzyme markers – These are biomarkers used to assess the function of specific organs in the body. For example, cardiac enzymes like troponin, lactate dehydrogenase and creatinine kinase are used to assess for myocardial infarction.

5. **End-of-life and palliative care** – End-of-life care is specialized care offered to terminally ill patients. Components of end-of-life care include planning, palliative care and advance directives.

   Palliative care is a component of end-of-life care. It involves the use of methods that improve the quality of life of terminally ill patients by providing relief from symptoms and addressing other emotional, psychological and spiritual needs. Components of active care include the provision of relief from pain and other distressing symptoms, affirmation of life and death as a normal process, neutrality and restraint from either hastening or postponing death, integration of the psychological and spiritual aspects of the patient's care, provision of support systems to patients and caregivers, an interdisciplinary approach and teamwork to meet the patient's needs and enhancement of the patient's quality of life.

6. **Pain prevention and management** – This includes the primary methods for preventing pain, such as position and posture and prompt and appropriate management of the underlying cause of pain. Pain management can be for acute pain, chronic pain syndromes or pain management as part of palliative care for terminally ill patients.

7. **Secondary prevention** – Secondary prevention methods are used to detect diseases early and prevent their progression. The principles of secondary prevention include:
   A. Early diagnosis and detection – Early diagnosis is possible when affected individuals have proper health-seeking behaviors, like screening, clinic visits and health education from experts.
   B. Early management – This includes the use of radiological, laboratory and clinical diagnostic tools in diagnosing disease and providing prompt treatment. Treatment options can be pharmacological, non-pharmacological or surgical.
   C. Follow-up and counseling – Follow-up is necessary to assess the quality of life of patients and for prognosis.

L. Multisystem – This makes up 10 percent of the test. Topics include:

1. **Acid-base disorders.** These include:
   A. Metabolic acidosis – This is caused primarily by reduced serum levels of bicarbonate (HCO_3-). This reduction causes the partial pressure of carbon dioxide to be reduced in compensation. As a result, there is either a marked reduction or slightly abnormal levels of pH. The two classes of metabolic acidosis are metabolic acidosis with a high anion gap and metabolic acidosis with a normal anion gap. The causes are ketonemia,

diabetic ketoacidosis, lactic acidosis, renal failure, drugs, malabsorption syndromes and others.

  B. Metabolic alkalosis – This disorder is caused by an increase in bicarbonate (HCO_3-). The partial pressure of carbon dioxide may or may not be increased. pH is typically high or nearly normal. Common causes of metabolic alkalosis include prolonged vomiting, use of diuretics, hypovolemia and hypokalemia. Sustained alkalosis is indicative of renal impairment. Clinical features include headaches, lethargy and tetany.

  C. Respiratory acidosis – This is caused by an increase in carbon dioxide with or without an increase in bicarbonate. The pH is usually low but may be near normal. It is caused by hypoventilation and is usually caused by the central nervous system, pulmonary or iatrogenic conditions.

  D. Respiratory alkalosis – This is primarily caused by a decrease in carbon dioxide, which leads to hyperventilation. There may be a decrease in bicarbonate, and pH may be high or near normal. Respiratory alkalosis can be acute or chronic. The chronic form is usually asymptomatic. Symptoms of acute alkalosis are confusion, cramps, syncope, paresthesia and lightheadedness.

2. **<u>Compartment syndrome</u>** – This occurs when pressure increases in tissues that are in a closed fascial space. Continued pressure can lead to ischemia. The first warning symptom of compartment syndrome is pain that is more than is warranted for the severity of the injury.

Causes of compartment syndrome include:

  A. Fractures
  B. Crush injuries
  C. Application of very tight casts, bandages and other tight circumferential devices
  D. Reperfusion injuries
  E. Other rare causes, including snake bites, burns, severe exercises and drug overdose.

Compartment syndrome typically occurs in the upper and lower extremities, but it can also happen in the abdomen and buttocks.

3. **<u>Distributive shock</u>** – Distributive shock is caused by the impaired distribution of intravascular volume in the face of normal circulating volume. It is caused by arterial or venous vasodilation. In distributive shock, there is either a bypassing of the capillary networks or a pooling of blood in the venous circulation and a consequent drop in cardiac output.

Causes of distributive shock include:

A. Anaphylactic shock
B. Septic shock
C. Severe spinal injury, usually above T4, which leads to neurogenic shock
D. Ingestion of certain drugs that cause massive vasodilation, like nitrates, opioids and adrenergic blockers.

4. **Failure to thrive (FTT)** – This is defined as a weight that is lower than the third to fifth percentile for age and sex, a progressive decrease in weight that is below the third to fifth percentile, or a decrease in the percentile rank of two major growth parameters in a short period. The causes of FTT may be medical or environmental. FTT can be organic, inorganic or mixed. Organic FTT is caused by an acute or chronic disease that affects food intake, absolution and metabolism, or increases energy requirements. In gerontology patients, organic causes acute cancers, terminal illness and chronic and infectious diseases.
Inorganic causes of FTT are neglect and other environmental factors. In gerontology, inorganic causes include eating disorders, poverty, mental disorders, substance abuse disorder, abuse and maltreatment.
Mixed FTT is characterized by an overlap of organic and inorganic causes.

5. **Fever of unknown origin (FUO)** – This is defined as a core temperature that is greater than or equal to 38.3°C and is not a result of a self-limiting illness or diseases with localized signs, or abnormalities that can be detected with a common test, like chest X-rays, blood cultures and urinalysis.

FUO is classified into:
A. Classic FUO – This is a fever that lasts more than three weeks with no identified cause after three days of being evaluated in the hospital or having three or more visits in the outpatient clinic.
B. Health-care-associated FUO – This is a fever in hospitalized acute care patients who do not have an ongoing or incubating infection on admission and whose diagnoses are uncertain after evaluation of more than three days.
C. Immune-deficient FUO – This is a fever in patients with immunodeficiency and neutropenia and/or whose diagnoses are uncertain after three days of proper evaluation.
D. HIV-related FUO – This is a fever that lasts for more than three weeks in HIV patients seen on an outpatient basis. It can also be described as a fever that lasts for more than three days in HIV patients who are admitted and whose diagnoses are uncertain after a thorough evaluation.

6. **Hypovolemic shock** – This shock is caused by a decrease in intravascular and circulating volume. A reduction in the preload causes a reduction in ventricular filling, cardiac output and stroke volume. Causes of hypovolemic shock include:
   A. Hemorrhagic shock caused by trauma
   B. Surgery
   C. Upper and lower GI bleeding
   D. Ruptured aneurysms
   E. Ectopic pregnancies, ovarian cysts and others.

Bleeding may be overt, as seen in hematemesis, or concealed, as seen in an ectopic pregnancy. Other causes of hypovolemic shock include burns, severe dehydration, hypernatremia, hyperpyrexia and severe gastroenteritis.

7. **Infectious diseases** – These include viral, bacterial, fungal, parasitic and hospital-acquired infections of all body systems.

8. **Morbid obesity** – This is a body mass index that is greater than or equal to 30 kg/m2. Causes of morbid obesity include:
   A. Genetic factors that regulate the consumption and metabolism of food, such as glucagon-like peptide 1 ([GLP-1), cholecystokinin (CCK) peptide YY (PYY), ghrelin, leptin, neuropeptide Y (NPY), agouti-related peptide (ARP), alpha-melanocyte-stimulating hormone (alpha-MSH)and others.
   B. It can also involve environmental factors, like portion sizes and energy expenditure.

The complications of morbid obesity are systemic. They include cardiovascular disorders, fatty liver, diabetes mellitus, cancers, cholelithiasis, cirrhosis, osteoarthritis, reproductive disorders, psychologic disorders and death. Treatment includes lifestyle modification, drugs and, in severe cases, bariatric surgery.

9. **Multisystem trauma** – These are injuries that involve more than one body system. Triage is important in managing patients with multisystem trauma.

10. **Pain** – Etiology, pathophysiology, assessment and management of acute pain and chronic pain syndromes. All these have been discussed in this chapter.

11. **Palliative care** – This has been discussed in section K.

12. **Sensory impairment** – Both cranial and spinal sensory nerve impairments, including their causes, risk factors, pathophysiology, clinical features and management.

13. **Substance withdrawal** – Physiological effects, symptoms and behavioral changes that occur when a substance is stopped or its intake is reduced. These effects are typically substance-specific. For it to be considered a substance withdrawal disorder, the syndrome must cause significant distress to the patient and/or impair functioning. Substance withdrawal does not include withdrawal symptoms that develop after a drug is used for its appropriate medical use and then withdrawn.

14. **Sepsis/septic shock and MODS** – Sepsis is a life-threatening dysfunction of organs that occurs when the body is overwhelmed by infection. It is a clinical syndrome characterized by reduced tissue perfusion and multiple organ failure. Common causes in immunocompetent patients include infection with gram-negative and gram-positive bacteria. Causes in patients with compromised immunity include atypical bacterial and fungal infections.
Septic shock is a consequence of sepsis. It is characterized by persistent hypotension, which is defined as the use of vasopressors to keep the mean arterial pressure above or equal to 65 mm Hg, a serum lactate level > 18 mg/dL even after the patient is resuscitated with intravenous fluids. Signs of septic shock include fever, oliguria hypotension and altered sensorium. Treatment involves aggressive resuscitation with antibiotics and fluids, supportive therapy, pus drainage and debridement of infected and dead tissue.

15. **Toxic ingestions** – General principles of managing poisons and other toxic ingestion include supportive care, use of activated charcoal for severe oral poisoning, use of dialysis, antidotes for specific poisonings and gastric emptying. Substances that are examples of toxic ingestions include alcohol, aspirin, vitamin supplements, over-the-counter drugs, heavy metals, adhesives, detergent, castor oil, bleach and others.

Chapter 3: Clinical Procedures

A. Cardiovascular Procedures – You are assessed on your ability to:

1. Insert arterial pressure catheters

1. Assess the anatomy of the preferred site. You can also use ultrasound guidance to assess the puncture site.
2. Assess the patient's risk of ischemia by doing the Allen Test.
3. Occlude the ulnar and radial arteries and encourage the patient to clench a fist tightly to exsanguinate it.
4. Encourage the patient to open his or her hand. This releases pressure from the radial artery. You will notice a quick return of color to the patient's hand. If the color return is more than ten seconds, do not cannulate the radial artery.
5. Dorsiflex the patient's wrist to about 60 degrees and use tape to attach the wrist to the short arm board.
6. Wear the appropriate PPE and observe asepsis.
7. Clean the venipuncture site with 2 percent chlorhexidine gluconate.

2. Insert a radial catheter

Option 1 – Blind method of placing the radial arterial line

1. Palpate the radial artery with your nondominant hand.
2. Insert the needle at a 30-degree angle to the surface of the skin. This should be congruent with the vessel's path with the dominant hand.
3. Puncture the vessel and note the return of blood.
4. Insert a guidewire to about 10 cm in depth.
5. Remove the needle while maintaining control of the guidewire and make a small incision adjacent to it.
6. Tunnel the catheter into the skin via the guidewire.
7. After a successful attempt, remove the guidewire and cover the catheter with a fingertip to avoid blood spills.
8. Quickly connect the arterial line transducer to the catheter and secure the arterial line.

Option 2 – Ultrasound-guided method of inserting a radial arterial line

1. Tunnel the needle through the vessel.
2. Use the ultrasound guidance to advance the tip of the needle into the artery.

3. Puncture the vessel and note blood pulsing into the dart chamber.
4. Slide the black tab on the catheter upwards to the needle.
5. Stabilize the needle and tunnel the catheter into the vessel via the wire.
6. Remove the dart device and leave the catheter in the vessel.
7. Cover the distal end of the catheter until the transducer is connected.
8. Suture the arterial line.

3. Insert a femoral arterial line

1. Identify the venipuncture site with an ultrasound. This is needed to cannulate the right vessel.
2. Use an anesthetic on the venipuncture site where indicated.
3. Use 1 to 2 ccs of saline for the procedure.
4. Connect the needle to the syringe and tunnel the needle while aspirating.
5. Use the ultrasound to advance the needle tip into the vessel.
6. Puncture the vessel and note the flow of pulsing scarlet red blood.
7. Keep the angle of the finder parallel to the skin.
8. Disconnect the syringe and insert the guidewire.
9. Remove the needle and confirm the position of the guidewire via ultrasound.
10. Make a skin incision that is adjacent to the guidewire and tunnel the catheter into the skin via the guidewire.
11. Remove the guidewire and cover the catheter with a fingertip to prevent air embolism. Connect the catheter to an arterial line transducer.
12. Secure the line with a suture.

4. Insert central venous catheters

Obtain consent before proceeding with the procedure. Having an assistant is helpful during the procedure.

1. Arrange your sterile supplies and position the patient with head down, if he or she can tolerate it, head facing away from the side of insertion.
2. Use an ultrasound area to define the point of venipuncture.
3. Observe asepsis by washing your hands and wearing a sterile gown and gloves.
4. Swab the area with the appropriate antiseptic and apply a sterile field.
5. Cover the ultrasound probe with a sterile sheath, use it to confirm the anatomy and insert the lidocaine.
6. As you wait for the lidocaine to work, flush and clamp all the lumens of the line except the Seldinger port.
7. Under ultrasound guidance, insert the Seldinger needle into the internal jugular vein.

8. When blood is aspirated, quickly remove the syringe and insert the Seldinger wire.
9. Anchor the inserted wire and remove the needle.
10. Make a small incision in the skin and tunnel the dilator over the wire.
11. Remove the dilator and tunnel the central line over the Seldinger wire.
12. Once the central line is in place, remove the wire and aspirate all lumens.
13. Re-clamp and cover all lumens with their appropriate clamps.
14. Suture the line, giving allowances for four points of fixation.
15. Dress with a clear dressing.

5. Interpret 12-lead ECGs

The 12-lead ECG has six limb leads that are placed on the arms and legs of the patient and six precordial leads that are placed on the anterior chest wall.

The limb leads are lead I, II, III, aVL, aVR and aVF. The precordial leads include leads V1, V2, V3, V4, V5 and V6. A normal ECG has waves, a complex, intervals and segments.

- Wave – This is the positive or negative deflection from a baseline that shows a specific electrical event. These waves include the P, Q, R, S, T and U waves.
- Complex – This is a combination of multiple waves that are grouped as a unit. The QRS complex is the only complex on an ECG.
- Point– The J point is the singular point in an ECG. It marks the end of the QRS complex and the beginning of the ST segment.
- Interval – This is the duration between two specific ECG events. It includes the PR, QRS, QT and RR intervals.
- Segment – This is the distance between two specific points on an ECG that are at the baseline amplitude. It includes the P, ST and TP segments.

The main parts of an ECG are the P wave, QRS complex and T wave. The P wave shows atrial depolarization. The QRS complex has the Q wave, R wave and S wave. It shows ventricular depolarization. The T wave, which is after the QRS complex, indicates repolarization.

6. Interpret ECG rhythms

The different ECG rhythms include:

A. Sinus rhythm – This is a regular rhythm that has normal Q-R-S, P, T deflections and intervals. Heart rate is 60 to 100 bpm at rest.

B. Sinus bradycardia – This is a sinus rhythm rate that is below 60 per minute in a gerontology patient.

C. Sinus tachycardia – This is a sinus rhythm that is more than 100 per minute in an adult. P waves are also present.

D. First-degree heart block – This is a sinus rhythm in which the PR interval lasts more than 0.2 seconds due to prolonged transmission from the atria to the ventricles.

E. Second-degree AV heart block – This includes Mobitz Type I (Wenckebach) or Mobitz Type II. In Mobitz Type I block, the PR interval lengthens progressively until the QRS complex drops. In Mobitz Type II, there is an intermittent drop in the QRS complex that is not typical of the Type I pattern. Also, in the Mobitz Type II block, there is no rapid progression to a complete heart block.

F. Third-degree heart block – This is called a complete heart block. There is a discontinuity between the P and QRS waves. The P-P intervals are usually regular, but they are not related to the QRS complexes.

G. Supraventricular tachycardia – There is a rapid atrial rhythm that has narrow QRS complexes. This rhythm comes above the bundle branches.

H. Atrial fibrillation – Afib (AF) is a common type of arrhythmia. There are absent waves before the QRS complex. The heart rate is also irregular.

I. Atrial flutter – This is a supraventricular arrhythmia. In this case, there is a saw-toothed flutter that is characteristically seen on the ECG that is in fact multiple P waves that appear for each of the QRS complexes.

J. Asystole – Another name for this arrhythmia is flat line. In this case, there is an absence of electrical activity on the cardiac monitor. The rhythm is responsive to defibrillation.

K. Ventricular tachycardia – Another name for this is Vtach (VT). In this arrhythmia, there are widened QRS complexes, absent P waves and an abnormal rate that is more than 100 per minute. This rhythm can quickly turn into ventricular fibrillation and death.

L. Ventricular fibrillation – Another name for this arrhythmia is Vfib (VF). In this arrhythmia, there is a chaotic wave pattern that has no pulse. VF may respond to electrical defibrillation.

7. Interpret echocardiograms – Echocardiograms are used to assess the heart's health, function and strength. Cardiac walls that are thicker than 1.5 cm are abnormal and can indicate high blood pressure or weak or damaged valves.

An echocardiogram is also used to measure the pumping action of the heart via the ventricular ejection fraction. The left ventricular ejection fraction is used to measure the proportion of blood pushed from the heart per beat. Echocardiograms give real-time pumping action of the heart, allowing health personnel to assess the force of contraction, the valves and the presence of structural defects.

8. Interpret hemodynamic values – This includes assessing hemodynamic values like:

A. Complete blood count – Components include hematocrit, platelet count and white blood cell count. This test can be used to assess and diagnose hematologic states, like anemia, polycythemia, thrombocytopenia, thrombocytosis, leukemia, leukopenia and others.
B. Erythrocyte sedimentation rate – This is used to assess and diagnose inflammatory conditions, like tuberculosis.
C. Coagulation profile – This includes clotting time, partial thromboplastin time and international normalized ratio. All these are used to assess and diagnose coagulopathies.
D. Peripheral blood films – These are used to assess the shape and number of blood cells, the color of red blood cells, the presence of inclusion bodies, parasites and others.

9. Interpret stress tests – Stress tests are used to assess the heart's capacity to handle stress. The patient is attached to a heart monitor and encouraged to exercise on a treadmill. The exercise is increased in intensity, and the heart rate, blood pressure, breathing and cardiac rhythm are measured both at work and at rest. Stress tests can diagnose coronary artery disease, cardiovascular causes of chest pain, shortness of breath and lightheadedness; determine safe levels of exercise and predict the risk of a heart attack.

10. Lead cardiopulmonary resuscitation team – The AG-ACNP may be involved in leading the cardiopulmonary resuscitation team for emergency and acute patients. This task requires rapid assessment and prioritization of acute patients.

11. Manage temporary transvenous pacemakers

A. Assess the patient's ability to tolerate the heart rhythm by monitoring the ECG, the patient's blood pressure, pulse, heart sounds, skin color, warmth, mental status and urinary output.
B. Assess the pacemaker for proper functioning – Do this by securing all connections and the generator box to the patient, checking the pacing threshold every 12 hours, replacing the battery generator, assessing and adjusting the sensitivity for understanding or oversensing.

C. Maintain electrical safety – Do this by assessing the wires for security and connectivity, keeping the insulation cover over uninsulated ends, using rubber gloves to handle exposed terminals, keeping unfounded equipment away from the patient and preventing liquid spills on the generator cables or insertion site.

D. Monitor for the insertion site for complications – On a daily basis assess for infection. On alternate days, change the dressing.

E. Assess patient's safety – Obtain informed consent before placing the pacemaker. Provide proper education to decrease anxiety, ensure proper positioning of patients to reduce tension on the external wires and generator, and use pain medications and sedatives where indicated.

12. Manage transcutaneous (external) pacemakers

Before inserting the pacemaker, the AG-ACNP must:

A. Explain the importance of the pacemaker, including its complications.
B. Order baseline EKG and blood tests.
C. Secure an IV access for fluids and medications.
D. Assess the baseline peripheral pulses, heart sounds and lung sounds.
E. Shave and prep the skin site for the generator.

After the procedure, the nurse must:

A. Monitor the patient for complications like pneumothorax, hemothorax, cardiac tamponade and perforation from the pacemaker lead.
B. Monitor the patient for lead dislodgement.
C. Monitor the ECG for signs of overspending, loss of pacing or loss of capture.
D. Provide adequate analgesia and other interventions when needed.
E. Assess the skin site for bleeding and/or infection.
F. Encourage the patient to be on bed rest for 12 hours and restrict movement of the affected arm for 12 to 24 hours.
G. Take precautions like avoiding heparin and aspirin for 48 hours.

Discharge instructions offered to the patient should include information and directions on:

A. How to place and operate the pacemaker, generator and leads.
B. Monitoring the site for bleeding and infection in the first week.
C. Not immersing the site in water for three days.
D. Reducing arm and shoulder activity of the affected arm to avoid dislodgement of new leads.

E. Avoiding playing contact sports and lifting heavy objects for two months after the surgery.
F. Contacting the physician if the patient feels fatigued or notices palpitations or recurrence of symptoms.
G. Checking radial pulse daily before rising from bed in the morning.
H. Carrying the pacemaker information at all times and wearing a MedicAlert bracelet.
I. Discussing all procedures with the cardiologist.

13. Perform cardiopulmonary resuscitation

How to perform hands-only CPR:

1. Put the heel of your dominant hand on the patient's sternum, then place your nondominant hand atop the other hand and interlace your fingers. Your shoulders must be above your hands.
2. Use your body as a weight and push down about five to six centimeters on the sternum.
3. With your hands on the chest, ease the compression so that the chest can return to the initial position.
4. Perform 100 to 120 compressions per minute.

14. Perform elective cardioversion – Elective cardioversion is typically done on an outpatient basis for patients with dysrhythmia. It can either be electrically or chemically induced. For electrical cardioversion, patients are sedated with IV sedatives. The nurse places electrodes on the patient's trunk and attaches these electrodes to a cardioversion machine. This machine monitors the patient's cardiac rhythm and then sends shock waves to stabilize the patient's cardiac rhythm. For chemical cardioversion, flecainide, dofetilide, propafenone, amiodarone or ibutilide are used for atrial fibrillation, while adenosine or verapamil is used for supraventricular tachycardia.

15. Perform emergency cardioversion – Emergency cardioversion is a life-saving procedure performed in the ER.

16. Perform ultrasound-guided diagnostic procedures – These include ultrasound-guided needle biopsy tests.

17. Perform ultrasound-guided therapeutic procedures – These include ultrasound-guided aspirations, drainage and catheterization.

B. Pulmonary Procedures – These include:

1. Initiate mechanical ventilation – Mechanical ventilators are assistive and life support equipment that is used to take over the breathing of patients with inefficient breathing. They deliver high oxygen to patients and filter out carbon dioxide. All these actions reduce the energy spent on breathing, allowing the patient's body to recover and heal. The nurse practitioner is expected to know the indications of a mechanical ventilator, which include severe heart disease, acute lung injury, coma, sepsis and septic shock, pneumonia, acute asthma, acute respiratory distress syndrome, respiratory muscle paralysis/weakness, chronic obstructive pulmonary disease, hypotension and others.

Mechanical ventilation can be invasive or noninvasive. Invasive ventilation includes endotracheal intubation, in which a tube is inserted through the patient's nose or throat, and tracheostomy, in which a tube is inserted into a hole made in the patient's throat. Invasive ventilation methods can also be used for bronchoscopy, in which the lung is examined with a bronchoscope that is inserted through the breathing tube. It can also be used for aspiration and administration of medications. Noninvasive ventilation includes continuous positive airway pressure (CPAP), which is used to deliver a steady and constant air pressure; adjustable positive airway pressure (APAP), which can alternate air pressure to suit the patient's breathing pattern; and bilevel positive airway pressure (BiPAP), which transmits air with different inhalation and exhalation pressures.

The nurse must be aware of the complications of mechanical ventilation, which include:

- A. Trauma to the upper airway
- B. Tooth avulsion
- C. Injury to the mouth, throat and vocal cords
- D. Injury to the trachea sinusitis
- E. Tracheal stenosis
- F. Ventilation-associated pneumonia
- G. Sepsis
- H. Lung injury
- I. Pneumothorax
- J. Oxygen toxicity and others.

2. Insert large-bore and small-bore chest tubes
- A. To begin, the AG-ACNP is expected to ensure the patient is stable.
- B. Confirm the purpose of the tube, whether it is for fluid or for air. This is necessary to ensure that the tube is appropriately placed for efficient drainage.

C. Proper positioning – Keep the patient's chest flat or ask the patient to flex forward to open up the intercostal spaces.
D. Landmarks – Identify the midaxillary line, nipple, tip of the scapula, twelfth rib and approximate line of the diaphragm.
E. Incision marks – Highlight the incision site with a pen before prepping and draping the skin.
F. Management of pain– Use general anesthesia for intubated and sleeping patients. For patients who are awake, you can use local anesthesia.
G. Dissection – Do a blunt dissection down the length of the thorax. Locate the superior part of the rib with your finger and be careful not to harm the neurovascular bundles in the intercostal space. The chest should be tunneled bluntly, using a curved Kelly clamp. Stabilize your dominant hand with your other hand to avoid putting the clamp too far into the chest and injuring the heart or lungs.
H. Dilation – Tunnel through the chest tube with a Kelly clamp, then secure the tube with a silk suture. Daily dressing of the tube should be done to avoid kinking.

3. Interpret pulmonary function tests

PFTs are used to diagnose respiratory diseases, evaluate the progression of lung disease, evaluate the efficacy of treatment and assess patients for the side effects of certain drugs.

The components of PFTs include:

A. Lung volumes – Components of lung volumes include tidal, expiratory, inspiratory and residual.
B. Tidal volume (TV) – Inspired or expired air at each normal breath when at rest.
C. Residual volume (RV) – Air remaining in the lungs at the end of exhalation at its maximum.
D. Vital capacity (VC) – Another name for this is forced vital capacity (FVC). It is the total air that is expired forcefully after inspiration at its maximum (IRV + TV + ERV).
E. Inspiratory reserve volume (IRV) – The maximum air on inspiration that is more than the tidal volume.
F. Expiratory reserve volume (ERV) – The expired air after tidal volume is expired.
G. Total lung capacity (TLC) – The maximum air in the lungs at inspiration. (IRV + TV + ERV + RV).
H. Functional residual capacity (FRC) – The air in the lungs after tidal volume is expired. (ERV + RV).

I. Spirometry and flow volume loops – Spirometry is used to record air that flows in and out of a patient's lungs. It is plotted against air that is inhaled and exhaled during various respiratory maneuvers.

These values are then compared with normal values established from reference patients according to size, age, gender and ethnicity. The most common measurements include forced vital capacity (FVC), forced expiratory volume in one second (FEV1) and the ratio of the two (FEV1/FVC), which is about 80 percent in normal patients. An FEV1/FVC that is less than 80 percent is suggestive of obstructive lung disease. Restrictive lung diseases have normal or increased FEV1/FVC.

Diffusing capacity is the measure of the ability of the lungs to transfer gas into the blood. Causes of low diffusing capacity include conditions that decrease the surface area for gas exchange (e.g., emphysema and pulmonary embolism), conditions that impair the blood's ability to accept gas (e.g., anemia), conditions that alter the permeability of the membrane or increase its thickness (e.g., pulmonary fibrosis).

The general approach to interpreting a pulmonary function test is as follows:

A. Determine if the FEV1/FVC ratio is low.
B. Determine if the FVC is low.
C. Confirm the pattern of restriction.
D. Grade the severity of the abnormality.
E. Determine if the obstructive defect is reversible.
F. Bronchoprovocation.
G. Establish differential diagnoses.
H. Compare the current PFT results with prior ones.

4. Manage mechanical ventilation – The AG-ACNP is responsible for creating nursing care plans for improving gaseous exchange, keeping the airway patent, preventing trauma, reducing anxiety and preventing cardiopulmonary complications. For example, management of ineffective clearance includes observing the color, odor, quantity and consistency of sputum to assess for infection; auscultating the lungs to assess for airway obstruction; monitoring the oxygen saturation before and after suctioning; assessing arterial blood gases for signs of respiratory compromise and assessing for peak airway pressures and airway resistance. Management modalities for ineffective airway clearance include turning the patient every two hours to mobilize secretions and reduce the risk of ventilator-associated pneumonia.

Commence airway suctioning as indicated when there are adventitious breath sounds and/or increased ventilatory pressure. Use closed in-line suction to decrease both the infection rate and hypoxia. Avoid saline instillation before suctioning.

Silence ventilator alarms during suctioning to decrease the frequency of false alarms and reduce stress to the patient. Administer adequate fluid intake for hydration and improve ciliary action to remove secretions. Administer pain medications as prescribed and as needed. Commence chest physiotherapy to lessen secretion and reduce the risk of pneumonia.

5. Order multimodal oxygen therapy – The AG-ACNP is expected to know when to order oxygen therapy and which oxygen delivery device to use. Oxygen should be administered to treat hypoxemia. However, it cannot treat breathlessness when there is no hypoxemia. A target oxygen saturation range should be used to guide the therapeutic administration of oxygen.

How to prescribe oxygen to guide therapeutic treatment:

A. Oxygen delivery devices – Oxygen is administered either via fixed performance or variable-performance devices.

B. Variable-performance devices – The quantity of delivered oxygen by these devices depends on the inspiratory volume of the patient, the amount of room air used during respiration, the oxygen flow rate and respiratory rate.

C. Reservoir mask – This device delivers non-humidified oxygen with about 60 to 85 percent concentrations. This device is ideal for patients who are very ill and need short-term oxygen supplementation.

D. Simple face mask – A simple face mask is to be used on a short-term basis. Oxygen is administered at 2 to 10 L/min. Face masks are inappropriate for patients with type 2 respiratory failure.

E. Nasal cannulae – Most patients can tolerate nasal cannulae because they are comfortable, so they can be used even when a patient is eating or talking. They are ideal for stable patients, to provide oxygen during meals and to provide nebulized therapy for those who need their oxygen controlled. Nasal cannulae are used in home settings. Flow rates that are more than 4 L/min can dry and irritate the nasal mucosa. They should be avoided if the patient has unstable type 2 respiratory failure.

F. Fixed-performance devices – These devices are used for patients who are likely to retain carbon dioxide.

G. Venturi valves – These are color-coded to identify the percentage of oxygen delivered. These percentages can be 24 percent, which is blue, and 60 percent, which is green. The minimum flow rate varies according to the oxygen-mask manufacturer. The AG-ACNP must confirm the recommended minimum rate for individual devices.

6. Order nasal/facial CPAP or BiPAP

Indications for use of a CPAP:

A. Maintaining airway patency in airway collapse as seen in patients with obstructive sleep apnea
B. Preterm infants with underdeveloped lungs and respiratory distress syndrome.
C. Hypoxia in infants with bronchiolitis, pneumonia and tracheomalacia.
D. Hypoxic respiratory failure, secondary to congestive heart failure.
E. Extubating patients who will benefit from positive airway pressure.

Contraindications:

A. A CPAP cannot be used for patients without spontaneous respiration (i.e., patients with a poor respiratory drive).
B. Uncooperative and extremely anxious patients
C. Unconscious patients
D. Trauma to the face
E. Air-leak syndrome
F. Severe vomiting
G. Copious secretions from the respiratory tract
H. COPD
I. Patients who have undergone facial, esophageal or gastric surgery.

7. Perform emergent intubation – The AG-ACNP should be able to perform emergency intubations in patients who are in respiratory and/or cardiac arrest.

8. Perform extubation – The AG-ACNP is responsible for extubating patients who no longer need a ventilator tube.

9. Perform rapid-sequence intubation (RSI) – Rapid sequence intubation is a form of emergency intubation where the patient is rapidly intubated to reduce the risk of aspiration. It is the fastest method of maintaining the emergent airway.

10. Remove the chest tube – The AG-ACNP is responsible for removing chest tubes from patients who no longer require such intervention.

C. Gastrointestinal Procedures

1. Insert small-bore feeding tubes

Indicated for patients with functional gastrointestinal tract but with an inability to ingest foods. Indications include:

A. Coma or depressed consciousness
B. Severe protein-energy malnutrition
C. Prolonged anorexia, burns and other illnesses that can cause metabolic stress
D. Head and neck trauma
E. Liver failure
F. Bowel preparation for surgery
G. Closure of enterocutaneous fistula
H. Intestinal resection
I. Malabsorption and others.

Small-caliber nasogastric tubes made of silicone or polyurethane are used for enteral feedings that are more than six weeks. For patients with nasal injuries or deformities, orogastric and other oroenteric tubes are used. For tube feedings that are greater than six weeks, a gastrostomy or jejunostomy tube is used. These tubes are placed endoscopically, radiologically or surgically. Jejunostomy tubes are used for patients with contraindications to gastrostomy, such as gastrectomy. Also, jejunostomy tubes are easily dislodged and should be used only on an inpatient basis.

How to pass a nasogastric tube:

1. Obtain informed consent from the patient. Wash hands and wear nonsterile gloves.
2. Position the patient upright with the head in a neutral position.
3. Measure the appropriate length of the tube by measuring the tube from the bridge of the nose to the earlobe and down to 5xm below the xiphisternum.
4. Lubricate the tip of the tube.
5. Use a local anesthetic spray in the oral cavity, aiming for the throat.
6. Inform the patient as you insert the tube through one of the nostrils.
7. Advance the tube gently through the nasopharynx. As you get to the esophagus, encourage the patient to drink some water or swallow saliva.
8. As soon as you get to the marked end of the tube, tape the free end to the nostril with a dressing.
9. Confirm placement of the tube by aspirating the gastric contents and test the aspirate with a litmus paper. A pH value that is less than four is indicative of correct placement.
10. If the aspiration is unsuccessful or the pH is greater than four, the patient will require a chest X-ray (CXR).

D. Renal/Genitourinary Procedures

Manage renal replacement therapies – This includes the management of patients on dialysis or with renal transplant.

1. Dialysis – Management plans for patients on dialysis include:

A. Monitoring fluid status – This includes monitoring the patient for fluid overload or dehydration. To reduce the risk for fluid overload/dehydration, maintain a strict fluid input and output chart, record the patient's weight serially and compare with the input and output chart. Assess the patency of the catheter and check for plugs, fibrin and kinks.

Also, assess the patient for abdominal distension, with associated diminished bowel sounds, constipation or change in stool consistency. Monitor vital signs like blood pressure and pulse and assess for pedal edema, bounding pulses and distension of neck veins. Also assess for features of electrolyte imbalance like muscle weakness, headaches, confusion, muscle cramps, confusion and disorientation.

B. Reducing the risk for injury/trauma – These risk factors include dislodgement of the catheter and consequent perforation of surrounding vessels and organs. This risk is applicable for both hemodialysis and peritoneal dialysis. To reduce these risks, encourage the emptying of the bladder before insertion of the peritoneal catheter, anchor the catheter with tape and restrain the patient's hands if indicated. Also, assess for signs of bowel perforation, which include the presence of feces in the dialysate effluent, a strong urge to defecate and severe watery diarrhea. Assess for a perforated bladder by noting the patient's urge to urinate or the production of large amounts of urine after the dialysis.

C. Reduce risk of infection – Infection risks include contamination of the catheter during insertion and periodic changing of the tubing and bags, contamination of the catheter insertion site by the skin flora and sterile peritonitis. To reduce the risk of infection, position the patient properly during dialysis by elevating the head of the bed to reduce tension on the diaphragm. Assess for signs of infection (i.e., fever and cloudy drainage of effluent). Observe aseptic techniques during catheter insertion and changing of dressings. Assess the color, odor and drainage at the insertion site. Obtain samples of blood and drainage effluent for microscopy and culture. Monitor the patient's BUN and commence antibiotic therapy as indicated.

D. Management of acute pain – The risk of acute pain includes catheter insertion, improper catheterization, peritonitis, infection, abdominal distension and infusion of cold or acidic dialysate. To reduce the risk of pain, assess the patient, noting the intensity using the pain scale and assessing for likely factors. Also, assess for pain that commences during inflow and the equilibration phase and assess for pain in the shoulder blade, which can be a referred pain from the diaphragm.

Elevate the head of the bed at intervals and turn the patient from side to side to relieve abdominal discomfort. Warm up the dialysate to body temperature before use to increase the rate of urea removal and prevent vasoconstriction. Use appropriate analgesics as indicated.

E. Integumentary Procedures

1. Administer local anesthetic – A local anesthetic is needed for performing procedures that require a local invasion of the skin. Examples of these procedures include skin biopsies, wound suturing and others.

How to administer local anesthetic:

1. Check the expiration date of the analgesic. Also, check the concentration of the anesthetic.
2. Disinfect your hands and put on a pair of sterile gloves.
3. Prep the skin by using the appropriate antiseptic.
4. Use a fine-bore needle for initial infiltration. You can use the static or continuous methods of infiltration.
   - Static method – insert the needle and aspirate to check that there is no return of blood. This confirms that you have not punctured a blood vessel.
   - Continuous method – insert the needle and inject the anesthetic continuously into the surrounding area.
5. Reduce the number of punctures by rotating the angle of the needle for maxim infiltration of the puncture site.
6. Confirm that the area is properly anesthetized before proceeding with the procedure. You can do so by pinching the area with a toothed forceps.

2. Incision and drainage of wounds – Incision and drainage are indicated for abscesses that are more than 5 mm. Untreated abscesses may slowly reabsorb into the tissue or spontaneously rupture. Rarely, there can be a deep extension into the subcutaneous tissue. This can cause sloughing and scarring.

How to perform an incision and drainage of an abscess:

1. Prepare the surface of the abscess by swabbing with chlorhexidine gluconate or povidone-iodine.
2. Drape the abscess with sterile towels and infiltrate with a local anesthetic. Be sure to use an appropriate amount of lidocaine and allow adequate time for it to take effect.
3. To avoid a downward rupture of the underlying tissue or rupturing, do not infiltrate into the abscess cavity.

4. Make a linear incision into the abscess. Be sure to create a widening for the incision for adequate drainage.
5. Wear the appropriate PPE in case of an upward rupture of the abscess.
6. Let the pus, blood and other purulent substances drain from the abscess. Probe into the abscess gently with curved hemostats to break up loculations. If indicated, manually express pus from the abscess.
7. Pack the abscess cavity with forceps.
8. Dress the wound in sterile gauze and tape.

3. Perform wound debridement – Debridement is the removal of dead, necrotic and devitalized tissues from a wound. There are different methods of debridement. They include:

A. Biological debridement – In this method, maggots are cultured in sterile environments and used to digest necrotic tissue. These sterile maggots are applied to the wound bed, and a dressing is used to keep the maggots in the wound.
B. Enzymatic debridement – Enzymatic agents are applied topically to liquefy and digest necrotic tissues. Antimicrobial agents are then used with collagenase to decrease the action of the enzymatic debridement. Enzymatic debridement is ideal for long-term patients, as it is not as painful as other methods.
C. Autolytic debridement – This is a very slow, almost painless method of debridement, and it is the most common method of debriding patients in long-term care settings. In this method, the body's enzymes digest the necrotic tissue. It is important to maintain moisture balance using dressings like hydrogels, hydrocolloids and transparent films.
D. Mechanical debridement – This can be done by irrigation, wet-to-dry dressings, hydrotherapy and the use of abraded techniques. Although this technique saves cost, it is painful and can damage healthy tissue. Also, wet-to-dry dressings are not ideal for long-term care.
E. Surgical sharp and conservative method – This is done with instruments like scalpels, curettes, rongeurs, scissors and forceps. Debridement depends on the depth of the devitalized tissue. This form of debridement is very aggressive and is performed in an operating room.

4. Prescribe wound care – The AG-ACNP is responsible for educating the patient on appropriate wound care for the rapid healing of a wound. Wound care includes adequate nutrition, mobilization, appropriate dressing and antibiotic use, blood sugar control, use of vitamin and mineral supplements and others.

5. Wounds – Sutures are inserted to hold body tissues together and facilitate wound healing. Sutures reduce dead space, support the wounds until they are healed and reduce the risk of infection and bleeding. The three types of suture techniques are as follows:

A. Interrupted suture – This is the most common technique used for suturing. The sutures are not connected but are done separately to reduce the risk of total breakdown of the suture. Also, individual stitches can be removed without compromising the wound closure. This suture takes longer and carries a risk of infection.

B. Continuous suture – In this technique, the stitches are connected all through the length of the wound. Although this technique is faster, it has a great risk of dehiscence if the suture material breaks. This technique is used for closing internal incisions.

C. Mattress sutures – Both horizontal and vertical mattress sutures are commonly used for skin closure because of their cosmetic effects. These sutures are used for skin incisions that require closure under tension and consequent eversion. These sutures are done using non-absorbable suture material.

F. Neurology Procedures

1. Care for the organ and tissue donor patient – This includes the provision of intense and critical care to potential donors who are brain dead and have advance directives to withdraw life support. It is important to provide critical care to these patients to improve organ perfusion and increase the chances of organ uptake.

A. Cardiovascular system – In the event of brain death, there is reflex hypertension and bradycardia to maintain the cerebral blood flow. Also, there is increased secretion and circulation of catecholamines, which cause vasoconstriction. All these mechanisms contribute to myocardial infarction and dysfunction. The goal of management is to maintain the blood pressure, optimize circulation and fluid and maintain oxygen perfusion into organs.

B. Respiratory system – There is a marked rise in pulmonary hydrostatic pressure that results in pulmonary edema. Respiratory management includes improved SpO_2 > 95%, $PaCO_2$ of 35 to 40 mmHg and pH of 7.35 to 45.

C. The endocrine system, stress and metabolic responses – Since endocrine functions are lost in brain death, it is empirical to commence hormone replacement therapy. Loss of function of the posterior pituitary leads to diabetes insipidus and consequent polyuria and hypernatremia. There is also decreased insulin function, leading to hyperglycemia. Also, temperature regulation is affected, causing initial hyperthermia, then hypothermia. Hypothermia increases the risk of acidosis, coagulopathies, arrhythmia and diuresis.

D. Systemic inflammatory response – SIRS is caused by inflammatory mediators from the brain, ischemic reperfusion injury and metabolic changes that occur during catecholamine activity.

Protocols for managing a donor patient include:

1. Keeping the core temperature to >35°C before the organ harvest. This can be done by using circulating hot air blankets, warming the intravenous fluids and adjusting the room temperature.
2. Since brain-dead patients are polyuric and dehydrated, crystalloids are used for fluid management. Crystalloid, like Ringer's lactate, is superior to normal saline because it does not cause hypochloremic acidosis.
3. Dopamine is the preferred inotrope in the event of hypotension, as it moderates the rate of injury and inflammation.
4. For ventilatory management, FiO2 should be kept to a minimum. Fluid resuscitation should be restrictive, and PEEP should be optimized.
5. Recommended hormone replacement is vasopressin, methylprednisolone, insulin and thyroxine.

2. Interpret cerebrospinal fluid results

2. Interpret cerebrospinal fluid results – This includes interpretation of biochemical, microbial and cytology tests done on cerebrospinal fluids. The following parameters are assessed in cerebrospinal fluid:

A. Opening pressure – Normal opening pressure is 10 to 100 mmH2O in younger children and 6 to 200 mmH2O from eight years. In obese patients, opening pressure can be as high as 250 mmH2O. Intracranial hypotension is an opening pressure that is less than 60 mmH2O. Opening pressure that is greater than 250 mmH2O is indicative of high intracranial pressure as found in meningitis, intracranial hemorrhage, tumors and other space-occupying lesions.

B. CSF color – Normal CSF is clear. Xanthochromic CSF is yellow, orange or pink discoloration of the CSF that is caused by hemolysis and consequent heme breakdown. Xanthochromic CSF can be seen in patients with subarachnoid hemorrhage, hyperbilirubinemia, or meningitis and when a traumatic tap is taken. The CSF of newborns is often xanthochromic because of their high levels of bilirubin and protein.

C. Cell differential – The CSF of a normal healthy adult has about 70 percent lymphocytes and 30 percent monocytes. A solitary eosinophil or PMN will be seen on rare occasions. It is not unusual to see several PMNs in a neonatal patient's CSF. Cell differentials are not enough to differentiate between bacterial and nonbacterial causes of meningitis. Lymphocytosis is seen in viral, tuberculosis and fungal causes of meningitis. The CSF of patients with bacterial meningitis is typically dominated by PMNs. Eosinophilic meningitis, which is 10 eosinophils per mm3, is indicative of parasitic meningitis. Other causes of eosinophilic meningitis include fungal, rickettsial and viral meningitis.

D. Protein level – Protein concentration is a very sensitive indicator of CNS pathology. CSF protein is elevated in infections, multiple sclerosis, Guillain-Barré syndrome, intracranial hemorrhage, malignancies and some use of drugs. Protein values can be falsely elevated by red blood cells in a traumatic tap.

E. Glucose level – The general rule is that CSF glucose is two-thirds of the serum glucose that is measured two to four hours before the CSF fluid is collected for analysis. Infections of the CNS can deplete the glucose levels in the CSF. However, glucose levels can be normal in viral infections. Also, normal glucose levels do not rule out a bacterial infection, as more than 50 percent of patients with bacterial meningitis will have a normal CSF glucose level. CSF glucose can also be lowered in chemical meningitis, subarachnoid hemorrhage and hypoglycemia. Elevated CSF glucose can be seen only in hyperglycemia.

F. Latex agglutination – This is used to diagnose bacterial antigen in the CSF. However, the sensitivity varies. Hemophilus influenzae has a sensitivity of 60 to 100 percent, but specificity is very low. While it may be useful for partially treated meningitis that yields negative cultures, it is not a routine test.

G. Polymerase chain reaction – PCR has high specificity and sensitivity for a lot of CNS infections. Although it is expensive, it can be used on small volumes of CSF, and it decreases the overall cost of diagnosis and treatment.

3. Perform brain-death testing – These clinical tests include:

A. Lack of response to noxious stimuli – Examples include pressure applied to the supraorbital ridge and nail beds. Spinally mediated reflexes are excluded.

B. Absent brainstem reflexes – These reflexes include pupillary light reflex, corneal reflex, oculocephalic reflex, ocular vestibular reflex, pharyngeal and laryngeal reflex and reflexes mediated by the trigeminal nerve.

C. Apnea test – This test assesses the integrity of the respiratory center of the brain stem when the blood levels of carbon dioxide are high. For this to be done, the patient is expected to be normothermic, hemodynamically stable with systolic pressure ≥100 mmHg, not on any paralytics or sedatives and have normal oxygenation (i.e., PaO2 ≥200 mmHg after 100% supplemental oxygenation). During this test, oxygen at a rate of 6 L/min is passed through a catheter that is at the carina after disconnection from the ventilator. The nurse assesses for respiration about eight to ten minutes after the ventilator is disconnected. A positive test is when there are absent respiratory efforts at a PaCO2 of 20 mmHg or 60 mmHg above the baseline in patients whose PaCO2 is elevated. The patient is confirmed as being brain dead after another test is done.

D. Other ancillary tests include CT angiography, transcranial Doppler and electroencephalography.

4. Perform lumbar puncture

A. Verify that there are no contraindications to the procedure. You may need to do a brain CT to exclude midline shift, active bleeding, cerebral edema and space-occupying lesions.
B. Obtain informed consent from the patient.
C. Do a neurologic exam to assess sensation, muscle strength and mobility of the upper and lower extremities.
D. Wash hands and observe asepsis when handling the lumbar puncture tray.
E. Put the patient in a lateral decubitus/fetal position, or sit the person upright and have him or her lean forward over a small table.
F. To locate the L3/L4 space, locate the superior iliac crests, palpating above and below to assess the widest space. Mark this location with the nail of your thumb, or use a pen or needle cap to make a small indentation.
G. Swab the skin with 2% chlorhexidine gluconate.
H. Set the LP tray and open the cerebrospinal fluid (CSF) CSF tubes, then drape the patient appropriately.
I. Anesthetize the area with 10 mls of 1% or 2% lidocaine.
J. Gently introduce the spinal needle at a cephalad angle. The bevel of the needle should face the longitudinal fibers to separate the fibers and not cut through them. The bevel of the needle should point upwards if the patient is in the lateral decubitus position. Point the needle to the left or the right if the patient is sitting up and leaning forward.
K. You will feel a popping sensation when you reach the subarachnoid space. Remove the needle and let the CSF drip out.
L. If the patient is in lateral decubitus, ask the person to stretch out his or her legs.
M. Attach the manometer to the end of the spinal needle and measure the opening pressure of the CSF.
N. Measure the opening pressure by attaching a sterile manometer to the end of the spinal needle.
O. Pour the CSF in the manometer into the first tube and then add 10 drops of CSF into the second, third and fourth tubes.
P. Withdraw the spinal needle and apply pressure with a sterile syringe. Reattach the obturator and withdraw it from the insertion site.
Q. Reassess the patient's neurologic status and document the procedure, including the number of attempts, opening and closing pressure and the total amount of CSF collected.

R. Encourage the patient to lie flat on his or her back and drink enough fluids to stay hydrated.

G. Behavioral Procedures

1. Use de-escalation techniques – These techniques are used to prevent crises that can erupt during the management of the acutely ill patient. Some of these techniques include using empathy, respecting personal space, setting limits, using nonthreatening and nonverbal language, ignoring challenging questions, focusing on feelings and avoiding confrontations.

2. Manage patients in restraints – This involves monitoring and evaluating the patient in a restraint. The patient's physical and mental status and response to the restraints are evaluated. The scope of monitoring must include physical statuses, like vital signs, skin integrity, hydration, nutrition, mobility, circulation, hygiene, elimination and comfort. It also includes psychological and emotional needs, like the patient's comfort, dignity and safety, as well as respect for the patient's rights

3. Ordering physical restraints – Physical restraints are manual methods, physical or mechanical devices, material and equipment attached to an individual's body that makes movement difficult. To order physical restraint, the AG-ACNP is required to include the reason for the restraint, the type of restraint to be used, how long the restraint is to be used and other instructions required according to a specific facility's policies.

H. Multisystem Procedures

1. Interpret diagnostic imaging – The AG-ACNP is expected to interpret results from imaging, like CT scans, MRIs, ultrasound scans, X-rays and others.

2. Prescribe durable medical equipment – The AG-ACNP is responsible for prescribing canes, wheelchairs, walkers, crutches and other durable medical equipment that is useful in improving a patient's quality of living.

3. Prescribe pharmaceutical interventions – This involves the prescription of drugs and other pharmaceutical agents needed for treatment and disease management.

4. Provide nonpharmacological interventions for pain – These include physical interventions, like massage, positioning, transcutaneous electrical nerve stimulation, acupuncture and progressive muscle relaxation. Also included are psychological interventions like guided imagery and biofeedback, mindfulness-based stress reduction, acceptance and commitment therapy and cognitive-behavioral therapy.

A. Massage – This involves kneading and rubbing the joints and muscles with the hands for relief of pain and tension. Massage relieves muscle tension by increasing blood and lymphatic circulation, decreases inflammation and edema, releases muscle spasm, stimulates the release of endorphins and releases signals that can override those of pain. Although it is not clear exactly how pain is reduced during massage, research has shown that massage can stimulate dopamine secretion that reduces the sensation of pain, improves mood and decreases depression and anxiety.

B. Positioning – This involves keeping the body in proper alignment so that stress and anxiety levels are reduced. Positioning can help reduce the risk of injuries, bed ulcers, muscle spasms and tension.

C. Hot and cold therapy – Warming can reduce pain, anxiety, nausea and heart rate in patients with chronic pain caused by colitis, cystitis, rectal trauma, cholecystitis and appendicitis.

   Warming therapy works by reducing the excitability of muscle spindle fibers. It also stimulates thermoreceptors in deep tissues and reduces pain mediated by the gate channels in the spinal cord. On the joints, warming reduces viscosity in synovial fluid, thereby increasing joint range and mobility.

   Warming is relatively affordable, is easy to perform and has few to no side effects. Cold therapy can increase the threshold of pain and decrease tissue swelling.

D. Acupuncture – In acupuncture, needles are inserted into certain parts of the body to stimulate nerves. These needles create small injuries that stimulate mild inflammatory responses, which can increase circulation, healing of wounds, modulation of pain and analgesia. Acupuncture is used to treat conditions like allergies, anxiety, chronic back pain, neck pain, shoulder pain and depression. It is also used to treat hypertension, morning sickness, migraines, strokes, insomnia and menstrual cramps.

E. Transcutaneous electrical nerve stimulation (TENS) – A TENS is an electrical device that uses electrical leads. These leads are attached to sticky pads that are placed on the inflamed area of the body. The TENS helps relieve pain by transmitting an electric impulse with a low voltage. These voltages, which have alternating impulses, activate large nerve fibers covered with myelin sheaths, thereby blocking the conduction of pain signals. The TENS reduces pain by stimulating the secretion of endorphins. TENS can be used on patients with chronic back, neuropathic and arthritic pain.

F. Progressive muscle relaxation – In this method, different muscles are tightened and relaxed to stimulate relief and comfort. This technique is used for patients with headaches, phantom limb pain, back pain and stress.

Chapter 4: Professional Caring and Ethical Practice

A. Advocacy/Moral Agency – This content makes up 3 percent of the test.

Core ACNP competencies

1. Advocate for improved access, quality and cost-effective health care.
2. Show an understanding of the interplay between practice and policy.
3. Demonstrate advocacy for policies that stand for equality, equity, cost and access.
4. Assess the legal, ethical and social factors that affect the development of health-care policy.
5. Contribute to health policy development.
6. Integrate the principles of ethics in making clinical decisions.
7. Evaluate the ethical implications of decisions.
8. Use ethically sound solutions to solve complex issues that are related to individuals, systems and populations.

AG-ACNP competencies

1. Use the standards of ethical and legal standards in handling health-care technology for adult-gerontology patients.
2. Recommend designs for clinical information systems, including age-appropriate clinical and social indicators.
3. Advocate for the use of the full scope of the AG-ACNP role.
4. Advocate for access to quality, cost-effective care within acute care health-care systems.
5. Advocate for the patient's and family's rights to health care decision-making, with full knowledge of the implications of ethical and legal standards.
6. Encourage patient and family decision-making in treatment options for complex acute, chronic and critical illness.

B. Caring Practices – This makes up 4 percent of the test.

Core ACNP competencies

1. Ability to form a nurse/patient relationship by using empathy, mutual respect and collaboration.
2. Ability to foster an environment of patient-centered care that ensures privacy, mutual trust, comfort, confidentiality and emotional support.

3. Ability to respect and protect the patient's right to autonomy in decision-making and negotiate a care plan that is mutually acceptable.

AG-ACNP competencies

1. Employ interventions that maintain psychological and physiological ability that is in keeping with the patient's age. These processes should be consistent with the aim of the patient's care.
2. Assess the patient's and family's ability to cope with and manage developmental transitions.
3. Initiate the discussion of sensitive issues with the patient, family and other caregivers.
4. Apply principles that can help in managing family stress and other forms of crises for patients and caregivers with critical, acute and chronic mental and physical illness.

C. Response to Diversity – This makes up 2 percent of the test.

Core ACNP competencies

1. Provide patient-centered care that recognizes the patient's cultural diversity and rights in autonomy and decision-making.
2. Integrate the patient's preferences in culture, spirituality, values, beliefs and other preferences.

AG-ACNP competencies

1. Develop and state views that have a positive impact on ageism and sexism in health-care policies and systems.
2. Demonstrate sensitivity to diversity in organizational cultures and populations.

D. Facilitation of Learning – This makes up 2 percent of the test.

Core ACNP competencies

1. Efficiently communicate both in oral and written formats.
2. Communicate evidence from inquiries to diverse audiences through the use of multiple modes.
3. Integrate appropriate technologies for knowledge management to improve health care.
4. Translate technical and scientific health information that is appropriate to the users.

5. Assess the patient's and caregiver's educational needs and provide effective and exclusive health care.
6. Coach the patient and caregiver for positive behavioral change.
7. Demonstrate skills in information literacy and complex decision-making.

AG-ACNP competencies

1. Contribute to the development of knowledge and improved care of the adult-gerontology population.
2. Provide guidance, consultation and mentorship to students, nurses and other health professionals in acute and critical care populations.
3. Collaborate with the patient, family and caregivers in developing educational interventions that are appropriate to the needs, values, development, cognition and literacy of the adult-gerontology patient.
4. Educate patients, families, caregivers and groups on the strategies for managing the interaction among normal development, aging and mental and physical disorders.
5. Adapt to teaching-learning methods that consider age, cognitive status, health literacy, readiness to learn, psychology, physiology and other factors.

E. Collaboration – This makes up 3 percent of the test.

Core ACNP practices

1. Provide leadership that can encourage collaboration with multiple stakeholders to improve health care.
2. Lead practice inquiry, either individually or in partnership with others.
3. Collaborate in planning for transitions across the continuum of care.

AG-ACNP competencies

1. Describe the current and evolving AG-ACNP role to other health-care providers and the public.
2. Develop advanced communication skills and processes for effective collaboration with formal and informal caregivers and professional staff for the achievement of optimal care outcomes for adult-gerontology patients.
3. Collaborate with intraprofessional and interprofessional teams and informal caregivers for the achievement of optimal patient outcomes during acute, critical and/or complex chronic illness.

F. Systems Thinking – This makes up 3 percent of the test.

Core ACNP competencies

1. Assume advanced and complex leadership roles that foster change.
2. Demonstrate reflective and critical thinking in leadership.
3. Advance practice through developing and implementing innovations that foster change.
4. Participate in activities and organizations that can affect advanced practices in nursing.
5. Evaluate the purpose of organizational structure, care processes, financing, marketing and policy decisions on the quality of health care.
6. Provide leadership in translating clinical knowledge to practice.
7. Contribute to the creation of health information systems that encourage cost-effective, safe and quality care.
8. Use technology systems that can capture data variables for evaluating nursing care.
9. Analyze the implications of health policies that affect various disciplines.
10. Apply the knowledge of organizational systems and practices in improving delivery of health care.
11. Create change by using a broad range of skills that include partnership, collaboration, negotiation and consensus-building.
12. Minimize risk and improve safety of patients, staff and other health-care providers at both system and individual levels.
13. Develop health-care policies and systems that can attend to the needs of populations, providers and stakeholders with diverse cultural needs.
14. Evaluate the impact of health care delivery on patients, providers, other stakeholders and the environment.
15. Analyze the organizational structure, resources and functions that can improve healthcare delivery.

AG-ACNP competencies

1. Coordinate health-care services for acute, critical and complex chronic illnesses.
2. Facilitate the highly complex structures that can improve health-care delivery to adult-gerontology patients.
3. Synthesize data collated from numerous sources, including technology and clinical knowledge, which are all necessary for clinical decisions that affect management, consultation and referral of all gerontology patients.
4. Improve the outcomes of clinical practice by using technology that can improve safety and monitor the outcomes of health-care delivery services.
5. Assess and evaluate the system barriers in technology that affect settings, health-care providers and geographic areas.

6. Assess the effect of external and internal health-care delivery systems on the health status of individuals and the population.
7. Determine the need for a transition to a different level of acute care or care environment after assessing the frailty, stability and acuity of the patient, including the need for supervision, assistance and monitoring.
8. Analyze the cost-effectiveness of high-acuity practice that accounts for risk and improvement of health care outcomes.
9. Initiate the transition of patients within health-care settings and across levels of acute care, including admissions, transfer and discharge.
10. Identify the processes, principles and regulations that are related to payer systems in the planning and delivery of complex health-care delivery services.
11. Describe the challenges to optimal complex care that are created by the competing priorities of patients, payers, providers and suppliers.
12. Encourage the use of safe and high-quality resources in promoting cost-effective care.
13. Analyze system barriers to acute care delivery and coordination.
14. Apply knowledge of the type and level of services that are provided across health care and community settings.
15. Help patients and caregivers understand complex health-care systems.
16. Collaborate with other professionals in tackling issues that concern the use of resources, quality of life and triage situations.
17. Organize comprehensive health care that cuts across diverse settings for adult-gerontology patients with acute, complex and chronic illnesses.

G. Clinical Inquiry – This makes up 4 percent of the test.

Core ACNP competencies
1. Critically analyze data to promote evidence-based nursing practice.
2. Integrate knowledge accumulated from science and humanities that are within the scope of the nursing practice.
3. Translate research, data and knowledge that can improve the outcomes and processes of nursing practice.
4. Use the best evidence available to continuously improve the quality of clinical practice.
5. Evaluate the relationships and influence of cost, quality, safety and access on health care.
6. Apply skills in peer review that can promote evidence-based practice and excellence.
7. Apply the various principles of nursing practice and interventions that can ensure quality nursing care.

8. Generate knowledge and clinical practice that can improve patient outcomes.
9. Apply research and investigative skills that can improve health outcomes.
10. Analyze clinical guidelines that can promote individualized practice.
11. Evaluate the impact of globalization on health-care policy development.

AG-ACNP competencies

1. Implement evidence-based interventions to promote safety and reduce risk in adult-gerontology patients.
2. Evaluate one's practice concerning the incorporation of evidence-based practice and leadership skills.
3. Participate in designing, evaluating and implementing standards of care that are based on clinical evidence and are appropriate to the patient's age and physiological and psychological needs.
4. Evaluate the risk-benefit ratio in adverse outcomes that can arise from under- or overtreatment.
5. Promote the delivery of evidence-based care for patients with complex acute, critical and chronic physical and mental illnesses.

Test 1: Questions

1. A 50-year-old woman presents to the ER with complaints of sudden chest pain that spreads to her back, diaphoresis, nausea and vomiting. On examination, her pulse is 90 bpm. BP on the right arm is 170/100, while BP on the left arm is 150/90. On auscultation, there is the presence of a diastolic murmur. Which of these diagnoses is most likely?

   A. Aortic aneurysm
   B. Aortic dissection
   C. STEMI
   D. NSTEMI

2. Patient K is a 55-year-old asthmatic who presents to the ER with complaints of crushing chest pain. His BMI on admission is 28 gh/m2. BP is 170/120 mmHg, and cardiac enzymes are markedly elevated, while ECG shows ST-segment elevation. The patient is noted to have diaphoresis and tachypnea at presentation. Which of these pharmacological therapies is contraindicated in this patient?

   A. Clopidogrel
   B. Low molecular weight heparin
   C. Propranolol
   D. Nitroglycerin

3. Which of these meal plans is suitable for a 45-year-old Jewish male admitted for a humeral fracture of the left upper arm?

   A. Spaghetti, meatballs and yogurt
   B. Rice, shrimp salad and orange juice
   C. Buttered toast and omelet
   D. Vegetable salad, shellfish and rice

4. A 52-year-old Muslim female is admitted for appendicitis. Her husband requests that only female nurses and physicians attend to her. Which of these responses is most appropriate?

   A. Explain that the hospital has a nondiscriminatory policy.
   B. Inform the managing team of the husband's request.
   C. Insist that the husband accept the team managing his wife.
   D. Write a report to the ER manager.

5. A non-English-speaking patient presents to the ER with a head injury. Which of these responses is most appropriate?

   A. Use sign language.
   B. Ask for the patient's caregiver.
   C. Request an interpreter.
   D. Speak slowly to the patient.

6. A 45-year-old Native American who just had an ORIF insists that he is not in pain and requires no pain relief. Which of these responses is most appropriate?

   A. Give the patient the analgesia as prescribed.
   B. Assess the patient for pain every 15 minutes.
   C. Respect the patient's cultural perception of pain.
   D. Use alternative pain therapy instead.

7. You are reassessing the clinical status of your patient, who just had a chest tube inserted for a massive pneumothorax. You notice the patient is in a prayer session with his church members and pastor. Which of these interventions is most appropriate?

   A. Come back later for the reassessment.
   B. Do your reassessment quietly and try not to disturb the session.
   C. Request permission to assess your patient.
   D. Ask the visiting group to wait in the waiting room.

8. Which of these meals is suitable for a Hindu patient who is admitted for a closed fracture of the right tibia?

   A. Tofu salad and basmati rice
   B. Chicken dhal curry
   C. Spaghetti and meatballs
   D. Shrimp fried rice

9. M is a 45-year-old immigrant from Ghana who is admitted for diabetic ketoacidosis secondary to undiagnosed diabetes mellitus. Which of these is M most likely to believe is the cause of her illness?

   A. Her illness is caused by stress.
   B. Her illness has a spiritual connection.
   C. Her illness is caused by an imbalance of yin and yang.
   D. Her illness is caused by a deficiency of insulin.

10. Patient M is a 65-year-old hypertensive diabetic who presents to the ER with complaints of chest pain, diaphoresis and difficulty breathing. His cardiac enzymes are markedly elevated; however, ECG shows no ST elevation. Significant findings on cardiac examination include bilateral crepitations on both basal lung fields. Which of these interventions is most appropriate?

    A. Immediate commencement of fibrinolytic
    B. Emergency angiography
    C. Angiography within 48 hours
    D. Emergency CABG

11. An 18-year-old female patient presents to the ER with complaints of breathlessness, chest pain and tenderness of the knees and elbows. Her temperature at presentation is 39°C, and an initial ECG shows a prolonged PR interval. A history of a throat infection is obtained. Which of these treatment options is not useful in this patient?

    A. Antibiotic therapy
    B. Methotrexate
    C. Prednisolone
    D. Aspirin

12. Patient M is a recovering IV drug user who has hyperpyrexia. There is a history of malaise and weight loss. On examination, he is noted to have painful red nodules underneath his toes. On cardiac examination, there is the presence of a regurgitant murmur. Which of these statements is correct?

    A. A definitive diagnosis requires echocardiography.
    B. A positive blood culture is a major diagnostic criterion.
    C. A history of intravenous drug use is a major diagnostic criterion.
    D. A predisposing heart condition is a minor diagnostic criterion.

13. A 45-year-old patient presents to the ER with chest pain, fatigue and dyspnea. The temperature on presentation is 38°C. ECG findings show an elevated ST segment. This patient complains of chest pain that worsens when he coughs. He finds relief by sitting up and leaning forward. Which of these is the most appropriate diagnosis?

    A. Aortic dissection
    B. Infective myocarditis
    C. Myocardial infarction
    D. Aortic aneurysm

14. A 65-year-old patient with dementia presents to the ER with his son. The son presents a legal document that grants him the legal right to make decisions on behalf of his father. Which of these accurately describes the son's relationship with his father?

    A. Guardian ad litem
    B. Health-care proxy
    C. Legal attorney
    D. Surrogate

15. Paramedics bring a 67-year-old male into the ER with hemorrhagic stroke. As the nurse on call, you notice that there are no relatives to give consent for an emergency craniotomy. Which of these steps is most appropriate?

    A. Step in as the patient's surrogate.
    B. Ask the paramedic to step in as a surrogate.
    C. Obtain an implied consent from the patient.
    D. Review the patient's medical records for an advance directive.

16. A 67-year-old male who is being managed for hepatic encephalopathy secondary to metastatic liver cancer has conflicting instructions in his living will and durable power of attorney. Which of these steps is most appropriate?

    A. Allow the health-care proxy to make the final decision.
    B. Leave the decision to the discretion of the attending physician.
    C. Review both documents for instructions on discrepancies.
    D. Contact the patient's lawyer for clarification.

17. An 18-year-old male is admitted to the ER with a penetrating injury to the chest following a traffic accident. On examination, you notice that the patient requires an emergency blood transfusion. His mother, however, insists that they are Jehovah's Witnesses. Which of these steps is most appropriate?

    A. Respect the mother's wishes.
    B. Obtain informed consent from the patient.
    C. Request the patient's durable power of attorney.
    D. Leave the decision to the attending surgeon.

18. Which of these is not a feature of informed consent?

    A. Disclosure of information
    B. Beneficence
    C. Competency of the patient
    D. Voluntariness

19. A 65-year-old female with Alzheimer's presents to the ER with dizziness, diaphoresis, fatigue and altered sensorium. A diagnosis of hypoglycemia is made. Her caregiver insists that the patient is a fussy eater. Which of these interventions is most appropriate?

    A. Monitor the patient for a few hours and then discharge her home.
    B. Encourage the patient to eat regularly.
    C. Prescribe vitamin supplements to boost appetite.
    D. Obtain a detailed history from the caregiver.

20. Which of these patients is unable to give informed consent?

    A. A 17-year-old married female
    B. A 35-year-old female with post-traumatic stress disorder
    C. A 65-year-old Asian immigrant who cannot speak English
    D. A 22-year-old male with opioid overdose

21. A patient is being managed in the ER for a penetrating trauma to the anterior chest wall. Chest X-ray shows blunting of the left costophrenic sulcus. Which of these findings is unlikely on a chest examination?

    A. Hyperresonance on the left border
    B. Hyporesonance on the left border
    C. Tracheal deviation to the right
    D. Respiratory rate of 35 cpm

22. M is a 24-year-old male who was rushed to the ER with a penetrating injury to the chest. Cardiovascular examination reveals chest pain, a harsh systolic murmur over the precordium, cold, clammy extremities and blood pressure asymmetry between the left and right upper limbs. An emergency chest X-ray reveals a widened mediastinum and deviation of the trachea to the right. Which of these diagnoses is most likely?

    A. Cardiac tamponade
    B. Aortic dissection
    C. Aortic disruption
    D. Hemothorax

23. A 25-year-old male presents to the ER with complaints of chest pain and difficulty breathing. There is a history of fainting following a strenuous workout session at the gym. On examination, a crescendo-decrescendo ejection murmur is heard at the right and left upper sternal border. Which of these is the most likely diagnosis?

    A. NSTEMI
    B. Aortic stenosis
    C. Aortic aneurysm
    D. Aortic dissection

24. Concerning the diagnosis above, which of these principles of management is correct?

    A. Confirmatory diagnosis is made by an ECG
    B. Chest X-ray findings include a widened mediastinum
    C. ECG changes may show LV hypertrophy
    D. Cardiac catheterization is the mainstay of treatment

25. You are describing the use of acupuncture as alternative therapy among Asian patients. Which of these models of qualitative research is most appropriate?

    A. Phenomenological model
    B. Ethnographic model
    C. Case study model
    D. Historical model

26. Nurse T's research paper is titled "Acute Management of Hypokalemia in a Patient with Anorexia Nervosa." What form of research is this?

    A. Correlational
    B. Quasi-experimental
    C. Case study
    D. Descriptive

27. You are conducting research that describes the effect of length of stay of surgical sutures and wound dehiscence. What model of research is this?

    A. Descriptive model
    B. Quasi-experimental model
    C. Correlational model
    D. Experimental model

28. Nurse O has a hypothesis that bedridden patients have a greater risk of decubitus ulcers. What form of hypothesis is this?

    A. Null hypothesis
    B. Simple hypothesis
    C. Complex hypothesis
    D. Logical hypothesis

29. You are researching the hypothesis that cigarette smoking can cause asthma in adolescents. Which of these research models is most appropriate?

    A. Experimental model
    B. Ethnographic model
    C. Correlational model
    D. Descriptive model

30. Which of these is an example of a nominal variable?

    A. Trade names of drugs used in research
    B. Blood pressure
    C. Ages of patients in a research study
    D. The total number of responses from a survey

31. You are conducting research that describes the action of calcium channel blockers on African American hypertensive patients. What type of variable is a calcium channel blocker?

    A. Independent, nominal
    B. Independent, ordinal
    C. Dependent, nominal
    D. Dependent, ordinal

32. A 55-year-old female patient presents to the ER with complaints of dyspnea, breathlessness, fatigue and chest pain. On examination, BP is 90/60 mmHg, PR is 120 bpm and RR is 40 cpm. During a chest examination, a pan systolic murmur is heard, and basal crepitations are in both lungs. What is the most likely cause of heart failure in this patient?

    A. Aortic stenosis
    B. Mitral regurgitation
    C. Mitral stenosis.
    D. Infective endocarditis

33. A 60-year-old female presents to the ER with cramping pain in both calves. There is a history of aggravation of pain during walking and pain relief on rest. On examination, BP is 150/100 mmHg and PR is 80 bpm. Both lower limbs appear dusky red on inspection. Which of these diagnostic tests is confirmatory?

    A. Ankle-brachial index
    B. Lipid profile
    C. Chest X-ray
    D. Echocardiography

34. A patient is admitted to the ER with meningitis. Significant findings on examination include a raised systolic pressure, wide pulse pressure and bradycardia. Which of these interventions is inappropriate?

    A. IV mannitol
    B. IV acetazolamide
    C. IV dexamethasone
    D. IV Ringer's lactate

35. A patient who is admitted to the ER is diagnosed with raised intracranial pressure. Which of the following is an appropriate form of treatment?

    A. Increase cerebral perfusion pressure
    B. Increase mean arterial pressure
    C. Increase cardiac output
    D. Increase PaO2

36. At the end of your shift, a colleague makes a pejorative statement about a patient to you. Which of these responses is most appropriate?

    A. Be tolerant of your colleague's response.
    B. Sharply rebuke your colleague.
    C. Inform others of your colleague's behavior.
    D. Confront your colleague openly and honestly.

37. Which of the following is the most appropriate method in handling disruptive patients from a low socioeconomic status?

    A. Use chemical/physical restraints.
    B. Refer such patients to another hospital setting.
    C. Establish a patient/nurse relationship.
    D. Avoid confrontations by refusing to attend to such patients.

38. You are discussing a sensitive issue with your patient. This discussion will have a great impact on his overall clinical condition. Which of these methods is the most appropriate way to involve the patient's family?

    A. Contact the family before speaking to the patient.
    B. Discuss the issue with the patient in front of his family.
    C. Exclude the family from the discussion.
    D. Discuss the issue with the family based on the wishes of the patient.

39. Your patient is an immigrant from Asia who has a large family that visits every day. Which of these methods is most appropriate in communicating information to the family?

    A. Appoint a representative who will relay the information.
    B. Arrange a weekly meeting to listen to the individual concerns of each of the family members.
    C. Allow the family to decide on a representative to relay the information.
    D. Allow the patient to decide on a representative to relay the information.

40. Which of these is the most appropriate method for reaching a consensus among the family members of a patient who is unable to give consent?

    A. Appoint the eldest family member.
    B. Appoint the patient's wife.
    C. Join the family in deciding on the most suitable representative.
    D. Allow the family to decide on a suitable representative.

41. Patient M has been recently diagnosed with type 2 diabetes. Which of these methods is most useful in helping him make permanent dietary changes?

    A. Schedule a follow-up visit with a dietician.
    B. Give the patient pamphlets on dietary modifications for diabetes.
    C. Encourage the patient to make healthy dietary choices.
    D. Counsel the patient to avoid high-calorie foods with low nutritive value.

42. Your hospital is located close to a deeply religious community with low socioeconomic status. How can you collaborate with the community in promoting health education?

    A. Organize outreach programs
    B. Offer free medical services
    C. Offer home services
    D. Give a health talk on television

43. Which of these features most supports a diagnosis of viral meningitis in a 35-year-old male admitted to the ER with fever, neck stiffness, vomiting and photophobia?

    A. Positive Brudzunski's sign
    B. Loss of deep tendon reflex
    C. Markedly elevated protein and PMNs and markedly decreased glucose
    D. Slightly elevated lymphocytes, normal glucose and normal opening pressure

44. A patient who has a chest tube for a large pleural effusion has the following results of his pleural fluid analysis: pale yellow fluid, pH 7.32, protein 24 g/L, specific gravity 1.011, LDH 140IU/L. Which of the following best describes this effusion?

    A. Exudate
    B. Transudate
    C. Hemorrhagic
    D. Chylous

45. A 55-year-old male presents to the ER with chronic cough, night sweats and fever. A history of exposure to a family member with chronic cough is obtained. The patient's PPD produces a 10 mm induration. Which of these interventions is most appropriate?

A. Acid-fast staining
B. Liver function test
C. Sputum culture and sensitivity
D. Airborne isolation

46. P is a 20-year-old motorcyclist who is admitted to the ER with penetrating trauma to the chest. At the presentation, he is delirious and complains of chest and abdominal pain. On examination, BP is 90/60 mmHg, PR is 100 bpm and respiratory rate is 40 cpm. The patient is noted to have distended jugular veins. Which of these echocardiography findings is most likely?

A. Collapse of the cardiac chambers
B. Dilatation of the superior vena cava
C. Left ventricular hypertrophy
D. Plethora of the spleen veins

47. Patient F is a 76-year-old hypertensive diabetic who presents to the ER with difficulty breathing, chest pain and restlessness. On examination, she has bilateral crepitations in the lungs. Her BP at presentation is 130/90 mmHg. Which of these findings is most likely to be found on echocardiography?

A. Massive dilation of the inferior vena cava
B. Dilated right ventricle with an increased ejection fraction
C. Dilated left ventricle with a decreased ejection fraction
D. Ventricular septal defect

48. A 45-year-old female who is admitted with diabetic ketoacidosis is about to be discharged with some written educational pamphlets. Which of these statements is accurate?

A. The reading level of most American adults is fifth to seventh grade.
B. Text-only content has more engagement and interaction.
C. Written materials should be supplemented with verbal instructions.
D. Written materials are not useful in patient education.

49. You are about to discharge a 25-year-old female who was admitted for complicated pyelonephritis. Which of the following information is false and should not be given to the patient?

   A. It is important to empty your bladder after sex to reduce the risk of a UTI.
   B. You should wipe from the front to the back after urinating.
   C. Cranberries are not effective in treating UTI.
   D. Wear breathable cotton underwear.

50. You are discharging a 45-year-old female who was admitted for an emergency appendectomy. Her discharge instructions should include information on:

   A. Rotavirus vaccination
   B. Mammography
   C. Contraception
   D. A high-fiber diet

51. Nurse M is a newly employed AG-ACNP. She is hired to work with cardiothoracic surgeons for emergency and elective surgeries. Which of the following best describes her position?

   A. Service-based practice model
   B. Population-based practice model
   C. Practice-based practice model
   D. Health-based practice model

52. Nurse T is hired to manage diabetic patients. Which of the following best describes her position?

   A. Service-based practice model
   B. Population-based practice model
   C. Practice-based practice model
   D. Health-based practice model

53. Nurse S is hired in a hospital setting to provide care to patients who present to the emergency room. Which of the following best explains her position?

   A. Service-based practice model
   B. Population-based practice model
   C. Practice-based practice model
   D. Health-based practice model

54. Which of the following patients has the greatest risk of cancer mortality?

    A. A 55-year-old male with advanced prostate cancer
    B. A 45-year-old female with advanced breast cancer
    C. A 45-year-old male with colorectal cancer
    D. A 40-year-old male with lung cancer

55. A 45-year-old patient presents to the ER with penetrating injury to the chest. Based on the symptoms, a diagnosis of cardiac tamponade is made. Which of the following clinical features is not a component of Beck's Triad?

    A. Hypotension
    B. Muffled heart sounds
    C. Bounding pulses
    D. Increased venous pressure

56. Which of the following is definitive management for a patient with cardiac tamponade?

    A. Pericardiotomy with thoracotomy
    B. Pericardiocentesis
    C. Thoracocentesis
    D. Thoracotomy

57. Patient R is a 35-year-old construction worker who presents to the ER with blunt trauma to the chest following a fall. On examination, he is found to have difficulty in breathing, localized chest pain and widespread petechiae on the middle and lower border of the left anterior chest wall. On inspection, he is seen to demonstrate a paradoxical breathing pattern. Which of the following features will not be seen on a chest X-ray?

    A. Three or more rib fractures
    B. Contusion of the lung
    C. Pleural effusion
    D. Cartilaginous disruption

58. M is a 65-year-old female who is admitted for hip replacement surgery. Which of the following principles is inappropriate in reducing the risk of pulmonary embolism?

    A. Anticoagulant
    B. Use of compression stockings
    C. Early mobilization
    D. Bi-hourly turning of the patient

59. A 65-year-old female is admitted to the ER with complaints of chest pain, difficulty breathing and restlessness. On examination, PR is 120 bpm, BP is 90/60 mmHg, Spo2 is 92% and RR is 40 cpm. A history of estrogen replacement therapy is collected. What is the definitive treatment?

   A. Antithrombotics
   B. Supplemental oxygen
   C. Percutaneous cardiac intervention
   D. Thoracocentesis

60. A homeless IV drug user is admitted to the ER with productive cough, chest pain, difficulty breathing and restlessness. Significant findings on examination include temperature 38°C, RR 40 cpm, HR 120 bpm and BP 100/60 mmHg. The patient's chest X-ray shows nodular opacities on both lung fields. All these are differential diagnoses except:

   A. Septic embolism
   B. Pneumonia
   C. Pulmonary embolism
   D. Infective endocarditis

61. A 25-year-old male is admitted to the ER with complaints of sudden onset of difficulty breathing, chest pain and restlessness. Significant findings on examination include BP 110/8 mmHg, RR 40 cpm, PR 100 bpm and SP02 86%. The patient is noted to have bluish discoloration of the fingers that does not improve upon oxygen supplementation. An emergency chest X-ray shows bilateral infiltration of the lung. Which of the following diagnoses is most appropriate?

   A. Lobar pneumonia
   B. Pneumothorax
   C. Acute respiratory distress syndrome
   D. Congestive heart failure

62. A 55-year-old patient who was admitted to the ER with shortness of breath, difficulty breathing and persistent hypoxemia has just been diagnosed with ARDS. Which of the following pathophysiologies is seen in ARDS?

   A. Elevated alveolar hydrostatic pressure
   B. Diffuse alveolar hemorrhage
   C. Severe bronchoconstriction
   D. Increased alveolar-capillary permeability

63. Patient M is a 22-year-old male who presents to the ER with difficulty breathing, chest pain, restlessness and bluish discoloration of his lips and mouth. Significant findings on examination include RR 40 cpm, HR 100 bpm, SP02 90%, BP 130/80 mmHg and digital clubbing. On chest examination, a holosystolic murmur is heard at the left sternal border. Which of the following best explains the pathophysiology of his respiratory failure?

A. Right-to-left shunting of blood
B. Inflammation of the lung parenchyma
C. Increased alveolar-capillary permeability
D. Metastatic spread.

64. You are about to perform a thoracostomy for a patient with a left-sided pneumothorax. Which of the following actions is inappropriate?

A. Mark the insertion site with a pen.
B. Properly prep the skin with chlorhexidine solution.
C. Inject lidocaine into the skin, subcutaneous tissue and rib periosteum.
D. Make a 1.5- to 2-centimeter skin incision in the fifth intercostal space, then bluntly dissect the intercostal tissue to the pleura.

65. You are performing a thoracocentesis for a patient with right-sided pleural effusion. Which of the following procedures is incorrect?

A. Percuss the area for hyporesonant sounds to assess the level of the effusion.
B. Select an incision point on the midclavicular line.
C. Prep the skin with 2% chlorhexidine solution.
D. Insert the thoracocentesis needle below the upper edge of the rib to avoid damage to the neurovascular bundles.

66. You are about to perform a thoracocentesis for a patient who presented with shortness of breath and nonpleuritic chest pain. Chest X-ray shows diffuse pleural thickening and blunted costophrenic angles. This patient has a history of chronic asbestos exposure. Which of the following is an unusual characteristic of the pleural aspirate?

A. Hemorrhagic
B. Viscous
C. Copious
D. Purulent

67. Patient M is a 15-year-old male admitted to the ER with chest tightness, shortness of breath, wheezing and coughing. On chest examination, there is tachycardia, crackles and stridor. Which of the following is diagnostic of asthma?

   A. An improvement in FEV1 of > 12% in response to bronchodilator treatment
   B. Patchy opacities of the lungs on chest X-ray
   C. An improvement in FEV1 of > 12% in response to corticosteroid treatment
   D. The flow-volume loop showing a reduction in air volume

68. Patient O is a 25-year-old known asthmatic who is admitted to the ER with complaints of chest tightness, shortness of breath and dizziness. On examination, there is tachycardia, tachypnea and wheezing. SPO2 in atmospheric oxygen is 87%. A diagnosis of acute exacerbation of asthma is made. Which of the following drugs is inappropriate?

   A. Nebulized salbutamol
   B. Magnesium sulfate
   C. Intravenous prednisolone
   D. Sodium cromoglycate

69. A 55-year-old patient presents to the ER with complaints of fatigue, shortness of breath and fainting spells. There is a history of chronic productive cough before presentation. Significant findings on examination include HR 100 bpm, RR 45 cpm and BP 100/60 mmHg. A chest examination reveals a barrel chest with hyperresonant percussion notes on both lung fields. Which of the following statements is correct?

   A. Diagnosis is confirmed by chest X-ray.
   B. This is a restrictive airway disease.
   C. Chest X-ray findings include massive pneumothorax.
   D. The patient is at risk of right ventricular failure.

70. All these are typical features of emphysema except:

   A. A barrel-shaped chest
   B. Pursed lip breathing
   C. Cachexia
   D. Pedal edema

71. A 55-year-old woman presents to the ER with complaints of shortness of breath and chest pain. A history of recent travel from Australia is obtained. Which of the following investigations is most appropriate?

   A. A chest X-ray
   B. An ECG
   C. An echocardiography
   D. A CT pulmonary angiography

72. A 65-year-old male is admitted to the ER with altered consciousness and seizures. On examination, PR is 120 bpm, fast and thready; BP is 100/60 mmHg; RR is 35 cpm. RBS is 600 mg/dL; osmolality is 325m Osm/L; serum ketones are 1.2mmol/L. Which of the following is the most appropriate diagnosis?

   A. Alcohol ketoacidosis
   B. Diabetic ketoacidosis
   C. Hyperglycemic hyperosmolar state
   D. Thyroid storm

73. Patient M is a 65-year-old male who is being managed for HHS in the ER. Which of the following treatment principles is inappropriate?

   A. Administration of IV 0.9% saline
   B. Administration of IM insulin
   C. Potassium replacement
   D. Dextrose infusion when the serum glucose is 250–300 mg/dL

74. Which of the following is not a typical feature of the patient with HHS?

   A. Severe dehydration
   B. Absent serum ketones
   C. Younger patient with type 1 diabetes mellitus
   D. Altered consciousness

75. A 45-year-old female presents to the ER with complaints of headaches, diaphoresis and palpitation. She complains that this is her third episode, each lasting for about 30 minutes. On examination, HR is 100 bpm, RR is 25 cpm and BP is 160/100 mmHg. Chest X-ray findings show a normal cardiac silhouette. Which of the following diagnoses is most appropriate?

A. Aortic dissection
B. Pheochromocytoma
C. Cushing syndrome
D. Hyperaldosteronism

76. Which of the following statements is false?

A. Urine-free metanephrine is more sensitive than plasma-free metanephrine.
B. Two or three normal urine-free metanephrine results when the patient is hypertensive rule out pheochromocytoma.
C. Chest and abdomen screening of the catecholamine test is positive.
D. There may be falsely elevated hematocrit levels.

77. A patient has just been diagnosed with pheochromocytoma in the ER. Which of the following principles of management is inappropriate?

A. Blood pressure control with beta and alpha-blockers is the treatment of choice.
B. Surgical removal is the treatment of choice.
C. Beta-blockers are used before alpha-blockers
D. Cortisol insufficiency is a complication of surgical removal.

78. A 65-year-old man is currently being managed for anemia secondary to ESRD. Which of the following is most likely to be seen in iron studies?

A. Increased serum ferritin, low transferrin saturation and increased TIBC
B. Increased serum ferritin, high transferrin saturation and decreased TIBC
C. Decreased serum ferritin, low transferrin saturation and decreased TIBC
D. Decreased serum ferritin, low transferrin saturation and increased TIBC

79. A 20-year-old African American man is admitted to the ER with complaints of dizziness, fatigue and pain in the feet, hands, back and thighs. On examination, he is found to be pale and icteric. The liver is palpable. However, the spleen is not. Which of the following statements is false?

A. Hydroxyurea may be useful.
B. Adequate hydration and analgesia are necessary.
C. Hemoglobin electrophoresis is diagnostic.
D. Splenomegaly is typically found in young adults.

80. A 25-year-old female is admitted to the ER with fatigue, dizziness and chest and abdominal pains. On examination, there is pallor, swelling of the left calf and hematuria. A history of previous occurrence during her last menstrual period is obtained. Which of the following diagnoses is appropriate?

A. Hereditary spherocytosis
B. Sickle cell anemia
C. Paroxysmal nocturnal hematuria
D. Porphyria

81. A 40-year-old female presents to the ER with fatigue and dizziness. Significant findings on examination are PR 100 bpm, fast and thready, and BP of 100/70 mmHg. She also has angular stomatitis and spoon-shaped nails. Which of the following cells are expected to be visible on peripheral blood film?

A. Microcytes
B. Blast cells
C. Macrocytes
D. Granulocytes

82. A 55-year-old woman presents to the ER with shortness of breath, chest pain and cyanosis. Significant findings include petechiae on the trunk, arms and lungs. Which of the following investigations is important for prompt treatment?

A. Platelet count
B. Hematocrit
C. D-dimer
D. INR

83. A 45-year-old female is currently being managed for rapidly evolving DIC secondary to septic shock. Which of the following management principles is inappropriate?

A. Aggressive treatment with antibiotics
B. Transfusion of cryoprecipitate
C. Platelet transfusion
D. Heparin therapy

84. A patient presents to the ER with increasing abdominal pain, vomiting, abdominal swelling and dizziness. On examination, there is abdominal tenderness and hyperactive bowel sounds. Which of the following diagnoses is most likely?

A. Peptic ulcer disease
B. Intestinal obstruction
C. Merkel's diverticulitis
D. Appendicitis

85. A patient who is in his second post-operative day for an emergency laparotomy and resection anastomosis complains of abdominal pain, nausea and vomiting. On examination, there is abdominal distension and hypoactive bowel sounds. Which of the following diagnoses is most likely?

A. Bowel obstruction
B. Intussusception
C. Paralytic ileus
D. Bowel infarction

86. Which of the following is not a test for acute appendicitis?

A. Rebound tenderness
B. Rovsing's sign
C. Obturator sign
D. Cullen's sign

87. Concerning the diagnosis of acute appendicitis, which of the following statements is true?

A. It is primarily diagnosed clinically.
B. A normal WBC count excludes diagnosis.
C. Rebound tenderness at the epigastrium is a typical feature.
D. A positive psoas sign is pain felt during the internal rotation of the flexed thigh.

88. A 35-year-old female is admitted to the ER with altered sensorium, vomiting and guarding. Significant findings on examination are HR 120 bpm, RR 35 cpm, BP 100/70 mmHg, abdominal tenderness and ecchymoses on the left and right lumbar regions. Which of the following diagnoses is most appropriate?

A. Acute appendicitis
B. Acute pancreatitis
C. Paralytic ileus
D. Acute cholecystitis

89. A 55-year-old male is admitted to the ER with altered sensorium, vomiting and guarding. Significant findings on examination are HR 120 bpm, RR 35 cpm, BP 100/70 mmHg, right-side tenderness and positive Murphy's sign. Which of the following diagnoses is most appropriate?

A. Acute appendicitis
B. Acute pancreatitis
C. Paralytic ileus
D. Acute cholecystitis

90. A 24-year-old female is being managed in the ER with massive hemorrhage secondary to a traffic accident. The patient's urine output has dropped significantly to 0.4 ml/kg/hour. Biochemical results are as follows: BUN/creatinine ratio 12, urine osmolality 445 mmol/kg, urine-specific gravity 1.009, urine sodium 45 mmol/L. Which of the following diagnoses is most likely?

A. Acute glomerulonephritis
B. Acute tubular necrosis
C. Prerenal azotemia
D. Chronic kidney disease

91. A patient is currently being managed for AKI secondary to aspirin poisoning. Which of the following is not an indication for hemodialysis?

A. Potassium > 6mmol/L
B. Uremic encephalopathy
C. Refractory pulmonary edema
D. BUN/creatinine ratio of 16

92. A 20-year-old patient is admitted with bilateral leg swelling, fast breathing and hematuria. On examination, BP is 130/100 mmHg and PR is 100 bpm. Dipstick urinalysis shows three pluses of red blood cells and protein. Which of the following principles of management is inappropriate?

A. Strict fluid input and output monitoring
B. Use of antihypertensives to control blood pressure
C. Transfusion of salt-poor albumin
D. Control of dietary protein

93. A 45-year-old woman is admitted to the ER with bilateral leg swelling, nausea, vomiting and flank pain. On examination, BP is 150/90mm Hg, and abdominopelvic USS reveals diminished cortico-medullary differentiation in the upper pole of the right kidney. Which of the following diagnoses is most likely?

A. Chronic glomerulonephritis
B. Acute glomerulonephritis
C. Focal segmental sclerosis
D. Minimal change disease.

94. A patient is being managed for chronic urinary retention secondary to benign prostatic hyperplasia. Which of the following is not a likely complication of obstructive uropathy?

A. Chronic glomerulonephritis
B. Hypertension
C. Posterior urethral valve
D. Hydronephrosis

95. A type 2 diabetes mellitus patient is admitted for DKA. Clinical examination reveals coexisting diabetic nephropathy. Which of the following statements is false?

A. Verapamil is renoprotective.
B. Glycated hemoglobin should be below 7.0.
C. Nifedipine is antiproteinuric.
D. ACEI is antiproteinuric.

96. A 45-year-old male presents to the ER with fatigue, dizziness, nausea and shortness of breath. On examination, he is found to be pale, with excoriations on both forearms. Biochemical results are as follows: urea 9 mmol/L, creatinine 600 umol/L, K6.5 mmol/L. Which of the following statements is false?

A. Definitive treatment is hemodialysis.
B. Iron deficiency anemia is a complication.
C. Ultrasound findings may reveal bilaterally contracted kidneys.
D. The definitive diagnosis is a renal biopsy.

97. A 36-year-old male presents with intense itching that is worse at night. Significant findings include erythematous papules on the scrotum, waistline, knees and in the web spaces of the fingers and toes. Which of the following treatments is most appropriate?

A. Ketoconazole
B. Permethrin
C. Retinoic acid
D. Loratidine

98. Which of the following interventions is inappropriate for a chronically bedridden patient with end-stage carcinoma?

A. Moisture barrier creams
B. Bi-hourly turning of the patient
C. Use of sheepskin
D. Use of linen sheets

99. A 22-year-old female presents to the ER with dysphagia, choking and altered voice. She also complains of drooping eyelids that worsen throughout the day. Sensation and deep tendon reflexes are normal. Which of the following diagnoses is most appropriate?

A. Multiple sclerosis
B. Guillain-Barré
C. Peripheral neuropathy
D. Myasthenia gravis

100. A known patient with myasthenia gravis is admitted to the ER with excess lacrimation, salivary secretion, diarrhea and proximal muscle weakness. On examination, HR is 120 bpm, and BP is 120/100 mmHg. Which of the following diagnoses is most likely?

    A. Myasthenic crisis
    B. Cholinergic crisis
    C. Parasympathetic crisis
    D. Amyotrophic lateral sclerosis

101. Which of the following is not a test for a patient who presents with clinical features of myasthenia gravis?

    A. Ice pack test
    B. Rest test
    C. Anticholinesterase test
    D. Electromyography

102. A patient is admitted to the ER with muscle stiffness and weakness of the lower and upper limbs. Significant findings on musculoskeletal exam reveal hyperactive reflexes and increased muscle tone. Which of the following diagnoses is most likely?

    A. Poliomyelitis
    B. Primary lateral sclerosis
    C. Amyotrophic lateral sclerosis
    D. Myasthenia gravis

103. Which of the following is not a typical feature of amyotrophic lateral sclerosis?

    A. Drooling
    B. Muscle atrophy
    C. Muscle spasticity
    D. Urinary incontinence

104. Which of the following is not a risk factor for Wernicke's encephalopathy?

    A. Refeeding syndrome
    B. AIDS
    C. Hyperemesis
    D. Vitamin B12 deficiency

105. A 57-year-old patient with a stroke has ptosis of the left eyelid. Significant findings on examination include miosis of the pupil and loss of sensation of pain and temperature on the left side of the face and right side of the body. On which part of the brain is the lesion most likely to be located?

A. Frontal cortex
B. Cerebellum
C. Pons
D. Medulla

106. A 22-year-old female is admitted to the ER for head injury secondary to a fall. Significant findings on examination include raccoon eyes, hemotympanum and otorrhea. Which of the following diagnoses is most likely?

A. Transtentorial herniation
B. Basilar skull fracture
C. Increased ICP
D. Subdural hematoma

107. A 55-year-old patient is admitted to the ER with hypertensive encephalopathy. On examination, eye opening is in response to pressure applied on the sternum; the patient says incomprehensible words to pain and responds with abnormal flexion to pain. What is his GCS score?

A. 8
B. 9
C. 7
D. 10

108. A patient is admitted to the ER with head trauma. Significant findings on examination include mydriasis of the left pupil, with concurrent paralysis of the oculomotor nerve and hemiparesis of the right side. Which of the following diagnoses is most appropriate?

A. Subfalcine herniation
B. Transtentorial herniation
C. Central herniation
D. Basilar skull fracture

109. A patient is admitted to the ER with traumatic brain injury secondary to a traffic accident. Significant findings on examination include headache, vomiting and nystagmus. Which of the following diagnoses is most likely?

    A. Transtentorial herniation
    B. Subfalcine herniation
    C. Tonsillar herniation
    D. Basilar skull fracture

110. A 22-year-old patient is admitted to the ER with a head injury following a traffic accident. Significant findings on examination include fixed dilation of the right pupil. Which cranial nerve is affected?

    A. Cranial nerve VII
    B. Cranial nerve II
    C. Cranial nerve III
    D. Cranial nerve V

111. An 80-year-old patient is admitted to the ER with confusion and drowsiness. Significant findings on examination include a GCS of 13 and a history of a fall three weeks ago. He currently takes oral warfarin for atrial fibrillation. Which of the following diagnoses is most likely?

    A. Subdural hemorrhage
    B. Extradural hemorrhage
    C. Cerebellar hemorrhage
    D. Epidural hemorrhage

112. A 45-year-old man has obsessive thoughts about germs on his hands. If he tries to stop washing his hands, he has palpitations. Which of the following treatments is appropriate?

    A. Sertraline
    B. Lithium
    C. Reserpine
    D. Bromocriptine

113. A 25-year-old female who is a recovering opioid addict is determined to quit, with the support of her husband and friends. Which of the following drugs is most appropriate?

A. Methadone
B. Lithium
C. Benzodiazepine
D. Sertraline

114. A 45-year-old male is placed on disulfiram for chronic alcoholism. Which of the following statements is false about the drug disulfiram?

A. It causes an accumulation of acetaldehyde in the liver.
B. It is suitable for patients with a high tendency to relapse.
C. Symptoms include facial flushing, headaches, tachycardia and sweating.
D. Patients are advised to avoid alcohol tinctures, elixirs and OTC cold and cough preparations.

115. A recovering alcoholic presents to the ER with ataxia, diaphoresis, altered consciousness and agitation. Significant findings on examination include PR of 100 bpm and temperature of 37.7°C. Which of the following diagnoses is most accurate?

A. Wernicke's encephalopathy
B. Korakoff's psychosis
C. Delirium tremens
D. Disulfiram reaction

116. A patient is brought into the ER with clinical features of benzodiazepine overdose. Which of the following features is most unlikely?

A. Miosis
B. Arrhythmia
C. Respiratory depression
D. Ataxia

117. A patient on chemotherapy for multiple myeloma develops anorexia, nausea and oliguria. Biochemical tests are as follows: Ca 5 mg/dL, uric acid 12 mg/dL, phosphate 7.5 mg/dL, potassium 6.5m Eq/L. Which of the following diagnoses is most appropriate?

    A. Chronic renal failure
    B. Paraneoplastic syndrome
    C. Tumor lysis syndrome
    D. Gout

118. A patient who is being managed for non-Hodgkin's lymphoma is currently being managed for tumor lysis syndrome. Which of the following interventions is unnecessary?

    A. Allopurinol
    B. IV normal saline
    C. Rasburicase
    D. Probenecid

119. Which of the following is not a cause of high anion gap metabolic acidosis?

    A. Diabetic ketoacidosis
    B. Aspirin poisoning
    C. Severe gastroenteritis
    D. ESRD

120. Which of the following pathophysiological tests describes Type A lactic acidosis?

    A. It occurs in normal tissue perfusion.
    B. It occurs in global tissue hypoperfusion.
    C. It is caused by an accumulation of byproducts of bacterial carbohydrate metabolism.
    D. It is caused by the impaired metabolism of amino acids.

121. A patient presents to the ER lethargic and with muscular fasciculations. Biochemical tests are as follows: HCO3 29 mmol/L, PCo2 42 mmHg, pH 7.5. There is a history of chronic use of laxatives and diuretics for weight loss. Which of the following interventions is appropriate?

    A. IV 0.9% normal saline
    B. Hyperbaric oxygen
    C. Ringer's lactate
    D. Hemodialysis

122. Which of the following is not a cause of respiratory acidosis?

   A. Opioid poisoning
   B. Severe asthma
   C. Severe poliomyelitis
   D. Anxiety disorder

123. A patient with a closed fracture of the left tibia complains of severe pain in the ankle. Significant findings on examination include exacerbation of pain on passive flexion of the toe. PR of the left dorsalis pedis artery is 60 bpm; pulse rate of the right dorsalis pedis artery is 80 bpm. Which of the following interventions is most appropriate?

   A. Splinting of the left leg
   B. Emergency fasciotomy
   C. IV analgesics
   D. IV normal saline

124. A patient presents to the ER with right shoulder pain after an episode of generalized seizure. On examination, the right arm is adducted and internally rotated. The X-ray of the right shoulder joint in the AP view reveals the ice-cream cone sign. Which of the following diagnoses is most appropriate?

   A. Anterior shoulder dislocation
   B. Inferior shoulder dislocation
   C. Posterior shoulder dislocation
   D. Shoulder subluxation

125. A patient is being managed for dislocation of the shoulder joint following a fall. Which of the following events is unlikely to be associated with the dislocation?

   A. Injuries to the brachial plexus
   B. Rotator cuff tears
   C. Fracture of the lesser tuberosity
   D. Injury to the axillary nerve

126. A 60-year-old presents to the ER with polydipsia and confusion. A history of breast cancer is obtained. Which of the following metabolic abnormalities is most likely?

A.   Hypocalcemia

B.   Hypercalcemia

C.   Hyperkalemia

D.   Hyperglycemia

127. A homeless male presents to the ER with complaints of early morning headaches and vomiting. Significant findings include ring-enhancing lesions on CT of the brain. Which of the following diagnoses is most likely?

A. CMV infection
B. Streptococcus infection
C. Toxoplasmosis
D. Aspergillosis

128. An 80-year-old female presents to the ER with agitation, shortness of breath and altered consciousness. There is a history of sore throat and cough before presentation. Significant findings on examination include GCS of 11 and hyporesonant sounds on the left hemithorax. Which of the following diagnoses is most likely?

A. Delirium tremens
B. Hypoglycemia
C. Toxic shock syndrome
D. Hypocalcemia

129. A 40-year-old male is admitted to the ER with weakness, fever and productive cough. Significant findings on examination include needle tracks on both arms, temp of 39°C, PR of 120 bpm, BP of 100/70 mmHg and RR of 35 cpm. A chest X-ray reveals bilateral cavitations on both lungs. Which of the following organisms is implicated?

A. Mycoplasma
B. Staphylococcus aureus
C. Chlamydia pneumoniae
D. Respiratory syncytial virus

130. A patient complains of diplopia while climbing the stairs. Which of the following nerves is affected?

   A. Abducent nerve
   B. Trochlear nerve
   C. Oculomotor nerve
   D. Trigeminal nerve

131. A patient presents to the ER with sudden onset of shortness of breath. Significant findings on examination include gray membranes in the tonsils and uvula. A history of travel to Cambodia is obtained. Which of the following organisms is most implicated?

   A. Candida albicans
   B. Hemophilus influenzae
   C. Diphtheria
   D. Streptococcus pneumoniae

132. You are to obtain blood samples from a patient who is suspected to be DUI. Which of the following steps is inappropriate?

   A. Swab the skin site with a tincture of iodine.
   B. Collect the sample in the gray-top tube.
   C. Select a visible straight vein.
   D. Remove the tourniquet after the needle is inserted.

133. You are to obtain informed consent from a patient who is booked for cardiac catheterization. Before signing the consent form, the patient is expected to have a full understanding of all these except:

   A. The process of cardiac catheterization
   B. The risks and benefits of cardiac catheterization
   C. Other alternatives to catheterization
   D. The cost of the procedure

134. Nurse T is part of the committee created to restructure the post-operative care given to patients with emergency abdominal surgeries, including when vital signs, laboratory tests and clinical assessments are to be completed and documented. Nurse T's committee is focused on improving which of the following?

   A. Critical pathway
   B. Quality planning
   C. Diagnosis-related group
   D. Multidisciplinary care

135. You are part of the committee that was created to restructure the steps taken for cardiopulmonary resuscitation on patients in the ER. Your committee is focused on improving which of the following?

    A. Quality control
    B. Critical pathway
    C. Multidisciplinary care
    D. Diagnosis-related group

136. You are collecting a sample for blood electrolytes, urea and creatinine. Which of the following steps is inappropriate?

    A. Collecting the right amount of sample
    B. Inverting the test tubes vigorously
    C. Swabbing with chlorhexidine gluconate
    D. Removing the tourniquet after inserting the needle

137. Nurse T is on a committee that has been set up to assess the rising cases of wound dehiscence among post-op patients. Part of this assessment is to assess the type of suture materials used for the patients. Which of the following is the committee focused on improving?

    A. Multidisciplinary care
    B. Quality control
    C. Critical pathway
    D. Diagnosis-related group

138. As the head of your nursing team, a rising case of needleprick injuries has been brought to your attention. Which of the following interventions is inappropriate?

    A. Review the Needlestick Safety and Prevention Act with all members of your team.
    B. Review the incident logbook.
    C. Screen all members of the team for bloodborne pathogens.
    D. Organize a phlebotomy training workshop.

139. A 65-year-old female is being managed post-op for a fracture of the femur. Which of the following interventions is most appropriate for helping her resume mobility?

    A. Elevating the affected limb with a pillow
    B. Using a wheelchair
    C. Using the overhead trapeze
    D. Using a cane

140. A 56-year-old male with head trauma secondary to a traffic accident is placed on nasogastric tube feeding. Which of the following interventions is most important when commencing a bolus enteral feed?

    A. Commence a high-protein feed
    B. Commence a high-calorie feed
    C. Monitor fluid intake and output
    D. Elevate the foot of the bed 30 degrees

141. A 56-year-old male who has been admitted to the ER with seizures secondary to suspected brain tumor complains of photophobia. Which of the following interventions is most appropriate?

    A. Transfer the patient to a private ward.
    B. Keep the screen closed to shut the light out.
    C. Prescribe an eye patch.
    D. Give IV diazepam to sedate the patient.

142. A 79-year-old male has just been diagnosed with Parkinson's disease. Which of the following interventions is inappropriate?

    A. A high-fiber diet
    B. Using Velcro
    C. Using elastic waistbands
    D. Using nonskid slippers

143. A 55-year-old female has just had emergency surgery for hemorrhagic stroke. Which of the following positions is most appropriate?

    A. Trendelenburg position
    B. Decubitus position
    C. Semi-Fowler's position
    D. High Fowler's position

144. A 45-year-old female who was admitted for left ventricular heart failure should be placed in what position?

    A. Recumbent
    B. Lithotomy
    C. High Fowler's
    D. Supine

145. A patient just had a thoracostomy for a massive right hemothorax. Which of the following interventions is inappropriate for his basic care and comfort?

    A. Monitor vital signs every 15 minutes for one hour.
    B. Place the patient in the semi-Fowler's position.
    C. Avoid lifting the drain above the level of the chest.
    D. Suction every two hours.

146. You are discharging a 25-year-old female who was admitted with anorexia nervosa. Which of the following specialists should she be first referred to?

    A. Dietician
    B. Psychiatrist
    C. Psychologist
    D. Endocrinologist

147. You are educating a group of middle-aged women about cancers of the reproductive system. Which of the following statements is false?

    A. Cervical cancer is predominant in non-sexually-active women.
    B. High progesterone is a risk for endometrial cancer.
    C. Old age is a risk for ovarian cancer.
    D. Early detection is key in the effective treatment of cancers.

148. A 25-year-old male presents to the ER with weakness, nausea, vomiting and abdominal pain. Significant findings on examination include slight jaundice and pain in the right hypochondrium and epigastrium. Hepatitis profile is as follows:

+ anti-HAV IgM

+ HBsAg

+ anti-HBcAg

+ anti-HBeAg

+HCV RNA

+ anti-HCV

Which of the following is most likely responsible for the patient's nausea and vomiting?

    A. Hepatitis A infection
    B. Hepatitis B infection
    C. Hepatitis C infection
    D. Hepatitis E infection

149. Which of the following investigations is appropriate for a patient who complains of frequency, hesitancy, dribbling and nocturia?

    A. PSA
    B. Prostate ultrasound
    C. Digital rectal examination
    D. Scrotal examination

150. A patient presents to the emergency room with a history of severe headaches following a fall in the bathroom. The patient is distressed because he cannot remember how he came to the emergency room. However, he can remember the events before the fall. This patient has which of the following?

    A. Anterograde amnesia
    B. Retrograde amnesia
    C. Mental block
    D. Personality disorder

Test 1: Answers and Explanations

1. (B) Aortic dissection.

Aortic dissection is a hypertensive emergency. It is caused by a tear in the tunica media of the aorta, allowing blood to flow within the tunica media. Symptoms include severe chest pain in the sternal region that radiates to the back, sweating, pallor, tachycardia, hypertension and focal neurologic deficits. An inter-arm blood pressure difference that is greater than 20 mmHg is an indicator of aortic dissection.

2. (C) Propranolol.

Propranolol is a beta-blocker routinely used for treating patients with unstable angina because it reduces heart rate, arterial pressure and general workload on the heart. However, it is contraindicated in asthmatic patients because it stimulates bronchiolar constriction and worsens pulmonary function in asthmatics.

3. (C) Buttered toast and omelet.

Kosher is the dietary regulation of Jewish individuals. This regulation forbids the consumption of pork and other non-hooved animals, as well as aquatic animals without fins and scales, like shrimp, oysters, clams and periwinkles. Also, the regulation forbids eating meat and dairy in the same meal. Therefore, buttered toast and an omelet is the most appropriate meal plan for this patient as it does not contravene any of his beliefs.

4. (B) Inform the managing team of the husband's request.

This response is most appropriate because it is important to inform the team of the caregiver's wishes rather than to make changes arbitrarily. All other options do not represent tolerance of diversity.

5. (C) Request an interpreter.

This response is most appropriate because it reduces the risk of misdiagnosis. The patient's caregiver may also be unable to speak fluent English. Using sign language and speaking English slowly is inappropriate.

6. (C) Respect the patient's cultural perception of pain.

Native American patients may not be as vocal or expressive with pain as European and American patients. It is appropriate to respect this patient's cultural perception of pain and wait watchfully until he requests intervention or until a clinical indication for it arises.

7. (C) Request permission to assess your patient.

This response is most appropriate. By obtaining consent, you make the visiting group aware of your presence. After obtaining consent, you may or may not ask that privacy be granted. It all depends on the clinical status of your patient. It is inappropriate to reschedule the assessment because this patient is unstable. It is also inappropriate to commence your assessment without introducing yourself and obtaining consent.

8. (A) Tofu salad and basmati rice.

Hindus are vegetarians because they believe that all life is sacred. Therefore the most suitable option is A because all other answer options include animal food sources.

9. (B) Her illness has a spiritual connection.

Because M is an immigrant from Africa, she may believe that her illness has a spiritual connection. African traditional religion teaches that most illnesses are related to imbalances between the physical body and spirits.

10. (B) Emergency angiography.

Emergency angiography is indicated for patients with complicated NSTEMI. From history, this patient has pulmonary edema secondary to left ventricular heart failure. Emergency angiography should be commenced. Option D is incorrect because although an emergency CABG may be beneficial to this patient, an angiography must first be done to ascertain if the MI is amenable to a PCI or a CABG.

11. (B) Methotrexate.

Methotrexate is an immunomodulator used in the treatment of rheumatoid arthritis. It is not appropriate for this patient, who has acute rheumatic fever. Salicylates are useful for the rapid relief of polyarthritis and carditis.

12. (D) A predisposing heart condition is a minor diagnostic criterion.

This patient should be evaluated for suspected infective endocarditis. The revised Duke's criteria for infective endocarditis are:

Major criteria: positive blood culture of typical infective endocarditis organisms, echocardiogram with oscillating intracardiac masses on the valves, single positive blood culture for Coxiella burnetti.

Minor criteria: predisposing heart condition or intravenous drug use, temperature greater than 38°C, vascular phenomena, immunological phenomena and positive blood culture that does not meet major criteria. Diagnosis is made with two major and zero minor criteria, or one major criterion and three minor criteria, zero major criteria and five minor criteria.

13. (B) Infective myocarditis.

This patient most likely has infective myocarditis. The patient has hyperpyrexia and shows symptoms of heart failure. Although his ECG findings are similar to that of myocardial infarction, chest pain in myocarditis is usually aggravated by thoracic motion and relieved when the patient sits up and leans forward.

14. (B) Health-care proxy.

A health-care proxy is someone who has been given the legal right to make health decisions for a patient who is incapacitated or unable to give consent. The document in which this authorization is given is called a durable power of attorney. Guardian ad litem is a title used to describe someone who has a legal right to be a guardian. Be aware that an attorney may not be a health-care proxy.

15. (D) Review the patient's medical records for an advance directive.

This answer is the most appropriate. Since the patient's caregiver cannot be identified, it is important to quickly review the patient's medical records for an advance directive. If a durable power of attorney is present, then the health-care proxy must be identified. If there is no advance directive, the AG-ACNP must determine a next of kin. If this is impossible, then a surrogate who is authorized by state law will be appointed.

16. (C) Review both documents for instructions on discrepancies.

Patients who have both a will and a durable power of attorney are encouraged to give instructions on conflicting instructions between the two documents. Most times, patients expressly state which document should be followed when the documents are conflicting. Other times, the documents are combined into the power of attorney.

17. (C) Request the patient's durable power of attorney.

This step is most appropriate because a durable power of attorney fact-checks the mother's claim and confirms the patient's consent to refuse a blood transfusion.

18. (B) Beneficence.

The components of informed consent include the decision capacity of the patient/surrogate, documentation of the consent, disclosure and competency. Beneficence is a component of medical ethics.

19. (D) Obtain a detailed history from the caregiver.

This patient is most likely a victim of elder abuse (neglect). It is important to obtain a detailed nutrition history from the caregiver to confirm your diagnosis. As soon as the diagnosis is confirmed, you should contact the elder abuse hotline immediately.

20. (D) A 22-year-old male with opioid overdose.

This patient has depressed cognition and awareness and is therefore ineligible to give informed consent. The 17-year-old is eligible to give informed consent because of her marital status. The 35-year-old and 65-year-old are eligible to give informed consent because they are not incapacitated in terms of cognition.

21. (B) Hyporesonance on the left border.

This patient has a hemothorax. The clinical features of hemothorax include chest pain, difficulty breathing, decreased breath sounds and hyporesonance on the affected side. Hyperresonance is a characteristic finding of pneumothorax, as opposed to hyporesonance.

22. (C) Aortic disruption.

The features of an aortic disruption include chest pain, a harsh systolic murmur over the precordium and asymmetric blood pressure and pulses between the left and right extremities. Although the features of an aortic dissection may overlap with that of an aortic disruption, a widened mediastinum is a characteristic finding for an aortic disruption.

23. (B) Aortic stenosis.

This patient most likely has aortic stenosis. The murmur in aortic stenosis is a characteristic crescendo-decrescendo murmur that is heard with the diaphragm of the stethoscope placed in the right and left upper sternal border.

24. (C) ECG changes may show LV hypertrophy.

In the principle of management of aortic stenosis, confirmatory diagnosis is by echocardiography, which shows a stenotic aortic valve. Chest X-ray findings will include calcification of the aortic cusps in cases of atherosclerosis. Cardiac catheterization is necessary to rule out a CAD, but it is not the mainstay of treatment. Aortic valve replacement may be beneficial.

25. (B) Ethnographic model.

This model of qualitative research focuses on cultural characteristics among a group of people. It focuses on how patients' religious and cultural beliefs impact their response to medical care such as acupuncture.

26. (C) Case study.

In the case study model, qualitative research is done on a single person to describe the actions and outcome of that single subject.

27. (D) Experimental model.

In the experimental model of quantitative research, the researcher attempts to use numerical data to describe the cause-and-effect relationship between two variables. In this model, the independent variable is identified and manipulated to determine its effect on the dependent variable.

28. (B) Simple hypothesis.

A simple hypothesis attempts to predict a relationship between two variables, usually a dependent variable and an independent variable.

29. (C) Correlational model.

In this model, the researcher attempts to observe and describe the relationship between two variables without manipulating the independent variable. In this case, the researcher will observe the effects of cigarette smoking in adolescents who are already smoking, without influencing the smoking habits of the adolescents.

30. (A) Trade names of drugs used in research.

A nominal variable is a form of categorical variable that is classified without rank or order. Examples include trade names of drugs, colors and other qualitative data.

31. (A) Independent, nominal.

The variable calcium channel blocker is an independent and nominal variable. This causative variable can be manipulated to elicit an effect on African American hypertensives. It is also a nominal variable because it is not categorized according to rank or order.

32. (B) Mitral regurgitation.

Pan systolic murmur is the cardinal sign of mitral regurgitation. It is heard at the apex of the heart with the diaphragm of the stethoscope placed when the patient is in the left lateral decubitus position.

33. (A) Ankle-brachial index.

This patient most likely has peripheral arterial disease. Diagnostic tests include an ankle-brachial index, which may be less than 0.90. Other confirmatory tests include Doppler ultrasonography and angiography.

34. (D) IV Ringer's lactate.

This patient has raised intracranial pressure as evidenced by the Cushing's triad: raised systolic pressure, widened pulse pressure and bradycardia. The treatment modalities include the use of IV mannitol and acetazolamide for osmotic diuresis, raising the foot of the bed to 30 degrees, IV dexamethasone and rapid treatment of the underlying cause. IV Ringer's lactate is not used to treat raised ICP.

35. (D) Increase PaO2.

The principles of treating increased intracranial pressure include decreasing PaCO2, increasing PaO2, decreasing blood flow and decreasing arterial blood pressure.

36. (D) Confront your colleague openly and honestly.

This response is most appropriate because it is assertive. It is important to confront your colleague about behaviors that can impair the functioning of the nursing team, but you must do it in a way that fosters collaboration and peaceful coexistence.

37. (C) Establish a patient/nurse relationship.

This is the most appropriate method because it helps the nurse build trust and reduce the risk of developing prejudice and bias, which may affect clinical judgment. Option A is incorrect because it is a form of battery. Options B and D are forms of prejudice and bias.

38. (D) Discuss the issue with the family based on the wishes of the patient.

This is the most appropriate response because your care is, first and foremost, patient-centered. The approach to collaborating with the family must be left to the discretion of the patient.

39. (C) Allow the family to decide on a representative to relay the information.

This method is most appropriate because it reduces the burden on the nurse and gives autonomy to the patient and his family.

40. (D) Allow the family to decide on the most suitable representative.

This response is most appropriate because it respects the autonomy of the family. All other options are inappropriate.

41. (A) Schedule a follow-up visit with a dietician.

This approach is most appropriate because follow-up visits to the dietician will help the patient make steady improvements in his dietary choices and objectively assess his progress and results.

42. (A) Organize outreach programs.

This is the most feasible, cost-effective and engaging option. Options B and C are not feasible, while Option D is not as engaging.

43. (D) Slightly elevated lymphocytes, normal glucose and normal opening pressure.

The findings that are suggestive of viral meningitis include slightly raised or normal lymphocytes, normal glucose, slightly elevated or normal protein and normal opening pressure. Option A is incorrect because it is a feature of meningitis regardless of the cause. Option C is incorrect because it is a biochemical profile of bacterial meningitis.

44. (B) Transudate.

Transudate effusions have protein that is less than 25 g/L, low or normal LDH, low specific gravity, low fibrin and low cell count. The macroscopic appearance of the fluid is clear and colorless.

45. (A) Acid-fast staining.

Based on the clinical history and positive tuberculin test, this patient has tuberculosis. Before the commencement of anti-Koch's therapy, confirmation must be obtained with an acid-fast stain of the sputum or gastric aspirate and a chest X-ray.

46. (A) Collapse of the cardiac chambers.

This patient has a cardiac tamponade caused by the thoracic injury. The echocardiography findings in a cardiac tamponade caused by a massive pericardial effusion are collapse of the cardiac chambers, particularly the right atrium and right ventricle. Other findings include dilatation of the IVC and a plethora of hepatic veins.

47. (C) Dilated left ventricle with a decreased ejection fraction.

This patient is in systolic heart failure. Echocardiography findings of heart failure caused by a systolic dysfunction are left ventricular dilatation with decreased ejection fraction.

48. (C) Written materials should be supplemented with verbal instructions.

This statement is accurate because verbal instructions are more engaging than written materials. Option A is false because the reading level of most American adults is eighth to ninth grade. Option B is incorrect because content that includes multicolored pictures engages readers better than solely text-based content. Option D is incorrect because written materials are very useful in promoting patient education.

49. (C) Cranberries are not effective in treating UTIs.

This statement is false because the effectiveness of cranberry juice in treating and preventing UTI is significant. Cranberry juice is said to contain compounds that can prevent the adherence of E. coli to the urethra and bladder mucosa. However, the effectiveness of these compounds is disputed. Also, their effectiveness is substantial compared to standard antibiotic therapy.

50. (B) Mammography.

This patient's age and sex put her at risk of having breast cancer. Yearly mammograms are indicated for women aged 40 and above.

51. (A) Service-based practice model.

The service-based practice model focuses on offering clinical management to specific patients who are then followed up with by a medical or surgical group.

52. (B) Population-based practice model.

In population-based practice models, AG-ACNPs are employed to manage patients with specific diseases (e.g., diabetes, thyroid disorders and others).

53. (C) Practice-based practice model.

In this model, AG-ACNPs are employed to provide care to patients in a particular unit of the hospital (e.g., patients in emergency rooms, labor wards, etc.)

54. (D) A 40-year-old male with lung cancer.

In the United States, the leading cause of cancer mortality in both sexes is lung cancer, followed by colon cancer, then rectal cancer. The leading cause of death in males is prostate cancer, while the leading cause of death in females is breast cancer.

55. (C) Bounding pulses.

The components of Beck's triad are muffled heart sounds, hypotension and increased venous pressure that is characterized by distended neck veins. Bounding pulses are not a component of the triad.

56. (A) Pericardiotomy with thoracotomy.

The definite treatment is thoracotomy with pericardiotomy or the creation of a pericardial window. Although pericardiocentesis is therapeutic, it is not a definitive treatment because blood in the pericardium is often clotted, and aspirations may yield negative results.

57. (D) Cartilaginous disruption.

This patient has a flail chest, which occurs when more than three ribs are fractured in the anterior chest wall and separate from the rib cage. Chest X-rays will show evidence of the fractured ribs, underlying pulmonary contusion and possible pleural effusion. However, cartilaginous disruption is not seen on X-rays.

58. (D) Bi-hourly turning of the patient.

This patient is at risk of venous stasis in the deep veins of the lower limbs. Option D is the correct answer because regular turning of the patient will not prevent pulmonary embolism.

59. (A) Antithrombotics.

This patient has features of pulmonary embolism. Estrogen therapy increases her chances of having a deep venous thrombosis in the lower limbs. Definitive treatment is the commencement of anticoagulant and antithrombotic therapy. Supplemental oxygen is a supportive treatment.

60. (C) Pulmonary embolism.

This patient has septicemia from IV drug use. Findings that support this diagnosis include a history of IV drug use, respiratory symptoms and chest X-ray findings. The features of pulmonary embolism include a history of deep venous thrombosis, chest tightness and Kerley B lines on a chest X-ray.

61. (C) Acute respiratory distress syndrome.

Although the symptoms of ARDS, pneumonia and CHF overlap, in ARDS there is no fluid overload, nor are there cardiogenic signs like heart murmurs. Most importantly, oxygen saturation does not improve even after the administration of supplemental oxygen. Also, chest X-ray findings of bilateral infiltration on both lungs are common in ARDS.

62. (D) Increased alveolar-capillary permeability.

In ARDS, there is an increased permeability of alveolar capillaries, which leads to a disruption in the production of surfactant and consequent collapse of the airways.

63. (A) Right-to-left shunting of blood.

This patient most likely has an atrial/ventricular septal defect of the heart. Increased pulmonary resistance causes a right-to-left shunting of blood, respiratory failure and hypoxia.

64. (D) Make a 1.5- to 2-centimeter skin incision in the fifth intercostal space, then bluntly dissect the intercostal tissue to the pleura.

This action is inappropriate because an incision should be made at the fourth intercostal space for a pneumothorax.

65. (D) Insert the thoracocentesis needle below the upper edge of the rib to avoid damage to the neurovascular bundles.

This statement is false because the needle must be inserted above the upper edge of the rib to avoid damage to the neurovascular bundles.

66. (D) Purulent.

This patient most likely has mesothelioma. Pleural aspirates are typically copious, hemorrhagic and viscous.

67. (A) An improvement in FEV1 of > 12% in response to bronchodilator treatment.

Option B is incorrect because chest X-ray findings of asthma include hyperinflation of lungs and mild atelectasis. Option D is incorrect because flow volume loops show reduced air entry.

68. (D) Sodium cromoglycate.

This is a mast cell stabilizer that prevents degranulation of unbound mast cells and their release of inflammatory mediators. It is used to prevent asthma attacks. Since it does not bind to already circulating mast cells, it is not useful for treating acute attacks of asthma.

69. (D) The patient is at risk of right ventricular failure.

This patient has COPD and obstructive airway disease. Option A is incorrect because the confirmatory test is a pulmonary function test. Option B is incorrect because this is an obstructive disease. Option C is incorrect because typical chest X-ray findings include a dome-shaped diaphragm, hyperinflated lungs and bullae.

70. (D) Pedal edema.

The clinical features of emphysema include cachexia, dyspnea, minimal cough, pursed-lip breathing, accessory muscle use, barrel-shaped chest and tachypnea. Pedal edema is typically seen in chronic bronchitis.

71. (D) CT pulmonary angiography.

This woman most likely has a pulmonary embolism caused by a DVT from venous stasis. A three-day flight from Australia to the United States puts her at risk for the condition.

72. (C) Hyperglycemic hyperosmolar state.

In a hyperglycemic hyperosmolar state, the patient presents with severe dehydration and serum blood glucose and osmolality that are higher than what is found in DKA. Also, compared to DKA, the patient may develop seizures and/or transient hemiplegia.

73. (B) Administration of IM insulin.

This statement is false because insulin is usually administered via an IV as a bolus rather than as an infusion. This is because the patient is severely dehydrated, so there will be poor absorption of the insulin if it is given IM.

74. (C) Younger patients with type 1 diabetes mellitus.

Option C is incorrect, as HHS is commonly seen in older patients with type 2 diabetes mellitus. In these patients, there is enough insulin to prevent the patient from going into ketoacidosis.

75. (B) Pheochromocytoma.

The classic features of pheochromocytoma include palpitations, headaches, diaphoresis and paroxysmal hypertension.

76. (A) Urine-free metanephrine is more sensitive than plasma-free metanephrine.

This statement is false because plasma-free metanephrine is more sensitive (99%) than urine-free metanephrine (95%).

77. (C) Beta-blockers are used before alpha-blockers.

This statement is false because unopposed beta-2-blockade can block beta-mediated vasodilation and create a paradoxical increase in blood pressure. Therefore, adequate alpha blockade must be administered before beta-blockade.

78. (D) Decreased serum ferritin, low transferrin saturation and increased TIBC.

This patient has iron-deficiency anemia. The features of iron studies in iron deficiency anemia are low hemoglobin, low serum iron, low ferritin, low transferrin saturation and increased high total iron-binding capacity.

79. (D) Splenomegaly is typically found in young adults.

This patient has sickle cell anemia, chronic hemolytic anemia that occurs almost exclusively in Blacks. Autosplenectomy and not splenomegaly is commonly seen in adults. Autosplenectomy is caused by splenic sequestration, repeated infarcts to the vasculature of the spleen and tissue atrophy.

80. (C) Paroxysmal nocturnal hematuria.

This is a cause of hemolytic anemia that is characterized by intravascular hemolysis, hemoglobinuria, arterial and venous thrombosis and pancytopenia. These features are paroxysmal and triggered by events like infections, vaccination and menstruation.

81. (C) Macrocytes.

This woman most likely has megaloblastic anemia caused by vitamin B12 or B9 deficiency. Although angular stomatitis is seen in iron-deficiency anemia, spoon-shaped nails are typically seen in megaloblastic anemia.

82. (C) D-dimer.

This woman most likely has pulmonary embolism and DIC. A D-dimer test is necessary to confirm a thrombotic episode and DIC.

83. (D) Heparin therapy.

Heparin therapy is not typically indicated for rapidly evolving DIC with bleeding or hemorrhagic shock. It is used for slowly evolving DIC and as prophylaxis treatment for patients with bleeding disorders.

84. (B) Intestinal obstruction.

The typical features of intestinal obstruction include abdominal pain, vomiting, abdominal distension, abdominal wall tenderness and hyperactive bowel sounds.

85. (C) Paralytic ileus.

The classic features of paralytic ileus include abdominal pain, nausea, vomiting and hypoactive bowel sounds.

86. (D) Cullen's sign.

This sign is used to clinically diagnose acute pancreatitis, not appendicitis.

87. (A) It is primarily diagnosed clinically.

Appendicitis is primarily diagnosed clinically, especially when the classic features are present. Radiological investigations are necessary for atypical and ambiguous clinical findings.

88. (B) Acute pancreatitis.

This patient has the classic features of acute pancreatitis: abdominal pain, guarding, positive Turner's sign, hypotension and tachypnea.

89. (D) Acute cholecystitis.

The clinical features of acute cholecystitis include right subcostal pain, nausea, vomiting and positive Murphy's sign, which is involuntary guarding of the upper abdominal muscles when the right upper quadrant is palpated during deep inspiration.

90. (B) Acute tubular necrosis.

This patient has ATN secondary to hypovolemic shock. Although the clinical features of ATN and prerenal azotemia may overlap, the biochemical findings are used to differentiate one from the other. Positive findings in ATN include BUN/creatinine ratio of 10 to 15.1, urine osmolality <450 mmol/kg, urine-specific gravity <1.010, urine sodium >40 mmol, among others.

91. (D) BUN/creatinine ratio of 16.

BUN and creatinine levels are not the best parameters for commencing hemodialysis. This is because the patient's clinical symptoms and state must be taken into consideration before commencing dialysis. For example, patients who are asymptomatic but have high BUN and creatinine levels are monitored, and hemodialysis is deferred until symptoms occur. This is done to reduce the risk of complications that arise from central venous catheters.

92. (C) Transfusion of salt-poor albumin.

This patient most likely has acute glomerulonephritis. Salt-poor albumin is not useful in this case because the edema is not caused by reduced oncotic pressure, but rather by increased hydrostatic pressure. Diuretics are more useful than albumin transfusion.

93. (A) Chronic glomerulonephritis.

The hallmark of chronic glomerulonephritis is the presence of tissue fibrosis that manifests on ultrasound as poor cortico-medullary differentiation. In this case, fibrosis has occurred, replacing the parenchyma in the renal cortex.

94. (C) Posterior urethral valve.

This statement is false because the posterior urethral valve is a cause of obstructive uropathy and not a complication. In the posterior urethral valve, an obstructing membrane causes vesicoureteral reflux and chronic retention of urine.

95. (C) Nifedipine is antiproteinuric.

This statement is false because nifedipine, amlodipine and felodipine are dihydropyridine calcium channel blockers. This class of calcium channel blockers has no antiproteinuric or renoprotective effects. However, drugs belonging to the non-dihydropyridine calcium channel blockers (diltiazem and verapamil) have antiproteinuric effects.

96. (A) Definitive treatment is hemodialysis.

This patient has chronic kidney disease with elevated urea, creatinine and potassium. Although hemodialysis will provide therapeutic relief from the elevated electrolytes, urea and creatinine, the definitive treatment is a renal transplant.

97. (B) Permethrin.

This patient has scabies, a parasitic infection of the skin. Classic features include an intense itching that is worse at night and papules on the waistline, scrotum, web spaces of the digits, axial and other folds of the skin. Treatment is with topical permethrin or lindane.

98. (D) Use of linen sheets.

This patient is at risk of developing pressure ulcers. The factors that increase the possibility of pressure ulcers include friction, shearing, moisture and pressure over bony prominences. Linen sheets can increase the risk of shearing and friction.

99. (D) Myasthenia gravis.

This patient has the classic symptoms of myasthenia gravis, which include ptosis that worsens throughout the day.

100. (B) Cholinergic crisis.

This patient has a cholinergic crisis caused by a high dose of anticholinesterase drugs. Mild symptoms resemble that of worsening myasthenia. However, in severe crises, there is increased lacrimation, salivary secretion, diarrhea and tachycardia.

101. (C) Anticholinesterase test.

In the anticholinesterase test, the patient is given a short-acting anticholinesterase-like edrophonium, and the patient's response to the drug is assessed. However, this test is not appropriate for a patient who presents with clinical features of myasthenia gravis because the test is not performed in the United States as edrophonium is no longer available in the country.

102. (B) Primary lateral sclerosis.

This patient has an upper motor neuron disease. Option B is a lower motor neuron disease; option C is a disease of both the lower and upper motor neurons and Option D is a disease of the neuromuscular junction.

103. (D) Urinary incontinence.

This is not a typical feature of amyotrophic lateral sclerosis. AML is a motor neuron disease characterized by progressive degeneration of the corticospinal tracts and the CNS. Typical features are muscle atrophy, fasciculations, muscle cramps, muscle weakness and weakness of the muscles of the mouth and throat. However, the cognition, sensory system, sexual functions, voluntary eye movement and actions of the urinary and anal sphincter are all spared.

104. (D) Vitamin B12 deficiency.

Wernicke encephalopathy is caused by impaired absorption or deficiency of thiamin in the face of continued consumption of carbohydrates. Risk factors include severe alcoholism, malnutrition, recurrent dialysis, hyperemesis, AIDS, starvation, cancer and others. Risk factors do not include vitamin B12 deficiency.

105. (D) Medulla.

This patient is suffering from lateral medullary syndrome, which is characterized by ipsilateral Horner syndrome and contralateral loss of pain and temperature sensation.

106. (B) Basilar skull fracture.

This patient has the classic features of basilar skull fracture, which are CSF rhinorrhea, CSF otorrhea, hemotympanum, Battle sign, raccoon eyes, loss of smell and loss of hearing.

107. (C) 7.

The patient's GCS is: eye opening – 2, verbal response – 2, motor response -3.

108. (B) Transtentorial herniation.

The features of transtentorial herniation, caused by a compression of the contralateral third cranial nerve and cerebral peduncle, are contralateral dilation of the pupil and paralysis of the oculomotor nerve and ipsilateral hemiparesis.

109. (C) Tonsillar herniation.

The features of tonsillar herniation include acute hydrocephalus that manifests as headache, vomiting, disconjugate eye movements, nystagmus, respiratory arrest and death.

110. (C) Cranial nerve III.

The oculomotor nerve is responsible for the pupillary light reflex.

111. (A) Subdural hemorrhage.

Subdural hemorrhage is commonly seen in the elderly. Also, subdural hemorrhage is not as severe as other forms of intracerebral hemorrhage. Extradural hemorrhage is highly unlikely in elderly patients.

112. (A) Sertraline.

This patient has OCD. Treatment includes the use of an SSRI like sertraline and cognitive-behavioral therapy.

113. (A) Methadone.

Methadone is the drug of choice for opioid abuse. Methadone is an opioid agonist-antagonist that suppresses withdrawal symptoms without producing a significant high for the recovering addicts.

114. (B) It is suitable for patients with a high tendency to relapse.

Disulfiram is effective for patients with a high motivation to overcome their addiction. Conversely, patients with a high tendency to relapse may risk drinking alcohol or be non-adherent to the prescription.

115. (C) Delirium tremens.

This patient has the classic features of delirium tremens, which are diaphoresis, ataxia, vestibular, tachycardia, agitation, fever and altered consciousness.

116. (B) Arrhythmia.

Overdose of anxiolytics and sedatives, like benzodiazepine, does not cause arrhythmia.

117. (C) Tumor lysis syndrome.

Tumor lysis syndrome occurs when there is a release of inflammatory mediators, cytokines and other intracellular components from lysed cancerous cells. It commonly occurs in patients with a large tumor burden, acute leukemia and non-Hodgkin's lymphomas. The significant findings of tumor lysis syndrome are hypocalcemia, hyperuricemia, hyperphosphatemia and hyperkalemia.

118. (D) Probenecid.

Although probenecid increases the excretion of uric acid, it is not indicated in the treatment of tumor lysis syndrome. This is because of the increased risk of nephrolithiasis in patients with a high risk of acute production of uric acid.

119. (C) Severe gastroenteritis.

This is a cause of normal anion gap metabolic acidosis. In high anion gap metabolic acidosis, there is decreased acid absorption/increased acid secretion and a concurrent decreased excretion of bicarbonate ions. In normal anion gap acidosis, there is increased reabsorption of chloride instead of bicarbonate.

120. (B) It occurs in global tissue hypoperfusion.

Type A lactic acidosis, the most serious form of lactic acidosis, occurs when there is an overproduction of lactic acid in ischemic tissues. It occurs primarily when there is global hypoperfusion of tissues, as seen in hypovolemic, cardiogenic and septic shock. Type B lactic acidosis occurs in normal perfusion, while Type D lactic acidosis, a rare form of lactic acidosis, occurs when there is an absorption of D-lactate, which is produced in the guts of patients who have had an intestinal resection.

121. (A) IV 0.9% normal saline.

This patient has metabolic alkalosis from excess loss of chloride ions. This form of alkalosis is chloride responsive. All other options are not useful to this patient. Hemodialysis may be needed when the pH is > 7.6.

122. (D) Anxiety disorder.

In respiratory acidosis, there is an accumulation of carbon dioxide due to a decreased respiratory rate, with or without a decrease in respiratory volume. This can be caused by impairment to the respiratory drive, impairment to the neuromuscular transmission and consequent weakness of the respiratory muscles or obstructive/restrictive airway diseases of the lungs. Anxiety disorder stimulates the respiratory drive, leading to hyperventilation and respiratory alkalosis.

123. (B) Emergency fasciotomy.

This patient has compartment syndrome, which is caused by increased pressure of tissues in a closed fascial space. An immediate fasciotomy is required to relieve the pressure and reduce the risk of tissue ischemia.

124. (C) Posterior shoulder dislocation.

Posterior shoulder dislocations are not as common as anterior shoulder dislocations. Causes include seizure, electrocution or electroconvulsive therapy done without muscle relaxants. Clinical features include adduction and internal rotation of the affected joint.

When the elbow is flexed, the joint may be passively rotated externally. The ice-cream cone/light bulb sign is a common finding on AP X-ray of the affected joint. Here, the head of the humerus is internally rotated. Therefore, the tuberosities do not project laterally. This makes the head of the humerus appear circular.

125. (C) Fracture of the lesser tuberosity.

Injuries that can be associated with a shoulder dislocation include injuries to the brachial plexus, rotator cuff tears, fracture to the greater tuberosity and injury to the axillary nerve.

126. (B) Hypercalcemia.

The most common cause of hypercalcemia is cancer and hyperparathyroidism. Features of hypercalcemia include constipation, anorexia, abdominal pain, ileus, polyuria, polydipsia and nocturia. More severe cases present as delirium, psychosis, stupor and coma.

127. (D) Aspergillosis.

Ring-enhancing masses in brain CT are classic features of CNS toxoplasmosis. Clinical features include headache, seizures, altered mental status, cranial nerve deficits and coma.

128. (C) Toxic shock syndrome.

This woman has delirium from a respiratory infection.

129. (B) Staphylococcus aureus.

This patient is an intravenous drug abuser. Implicated organisms are staphylococcus aureus, which presents as cavitating lesions on a chest X-ray.

130. (B) Trochlear nerve.

The trochlear nerve innervates the superior oblique, which is responsible for downward gaze. Palsy of the oculomotor nerve can cause double vision because it innervates the inferior rectus, medial and superior recti muscles.

131. (C) Diphtheria.

Features that support this diagnosis include a history of recent travel to Cambodia, gray membrane in the tonsils and uvula, and shortness of breath.

132. (A) Swab the skin site with tincture of iodine.

This step is inappropriate because the skin site must be swabbed with a non-alcohol-based antiseptic, like chlorhexidine gluconate or povidone-iodine.

133. (D) The cost of the procedure.

The patient does not need this information before signing the consent form. The information needed includes the process and purpose of the procedure, the risks and benefits and other alternatives.

134. (A) Critical pathway.

A critical pathway is a flow chart of activities that organize the care delivered by health workers. It includes patient activities and the time these activities should be completed.

135. (B) Critical pathway.

A critical pathway is a flow chart of activities that organizes the care delivered by health workers. It includes patient activities and the time these activities should be completed.

136. (B) Inverting the test tubes vigorously.

Vigorous inversion of the tubes may cause hemolysis. This can cause false-positive results of hyperkalemia and anemia. The tubes should be gently inverted about eight times for adequate mixing with the anticoagulant.

137. (B) Quality control.

In health care, quality control measures are undertaken to ensure that standardized practices and principles are used to ensure maximum safety to both patients and health workers.

138. (C) Screen all members of the team for bloodborne pathogens.

This action is inappropriate because it is expected that nurses with needlestick injury should have logged their incident in the logbook, along with the action taken. Screening all members of the team for bloodborne pathogens does not show that the pathogens were transmitted through needlestick injuries.

139. (C) Using the overhead trapeze.

This is the most appropriate intervention because the trapeze helps the woman strengthen her upper body in preparation for mobility. Also, compared to the wheelchair and cane, it is the safest option for improving blood circulation and mobility in this patient.

140. (C) Monitor fluid intake and output.

Enteral feedings are hyperosmolar agents that can cause osmotic diuresis in this patient and increase both intravascular and intracranial pressure. It is important to measure fluid intake and output. The head of the bed, not the foot of the bed, is raised 30 degrees.

141. (C) Prescribe an eye patch.

An eye patch is the most appropriate response. Moving the patient to a private ward or screening the patient is not appropriate because this patient is highly unstable. Sedating him with IV diazepam can be deemed a chemical restraint and assault.

142. (D) Using nonskid slippers.

This intervention is inappropriate because slippers of any kind can increase the risk of trips and falls. Patients with Parkinson's are encouraged to wear well-fitting, nonskid shoes to reduce the risk of trips and falls.

143. (C) Semi-Fowler's position.

In this position, the patient is placed with her head elevated to an angle of about 30 degrees. This angle helps improve blood drainage from the head and reduces cerebral edema.

144. (C) High Fowler's.

The high Fowler's position is also called the cardiac position. This position helps relieve the symptoms of pulmonary congestion by allowing gravity to move the fluid to the base of the lungs.

145. (D) Suction every two hours.

Frequent suctioning will do more harm than good. It will cause discomfort to the patient, and it can traumatize tissues and cause air leak syndromes. Suctioning should be done only when indicated.

146. (B) Psychiatrist.

Anorexia nervosa is an eating disorder that must be managed by a psychiatrist. After the psychiatrist's evaluation, the patient is then comanaged by a dietician, endocrinologist and other health specialists.

147. (A) Cervical cancer is predominant in non-sexually-active women.

This statement is false because women who are not sexually active have a very low risk of having cervical cancer. This is because they have a low risk of exposure to the carcinogenic strains of HPV, and they also have little or no exposure to combined oral contraceptives.

148. (A) Hepatitis A infection.

Based on the results, this patient has an acute infection with hepatitis A and chronic hepatitis B and C infections. The acute infection with hepatitis A is responsible for the gastroenteric symptoms.

149. (C) Digital rectal examination.

This patient has a bladder outlet obstruction, which may be caused by benign prostatic hyperplasia or prostate cancer. A digital rectal examination is an appropriate answer because it gives the nurse practitioner insight into the nature of the mass, including its size, consistency, texture and attachment to surrounding structures. Option A is incorrect because a PSA is not specific in diagnosing prostatic cancer. Option B is incorrect because although a prostate ultrasound is important, it must be done after the digital rectal examination.

150. (A) Anterograde amnesia.

Anterograde amnesia is an inability to create new memories after the event that caused the amnesia. This causes a partial or complete inability to recall the recent past. However, long-term memories from before the event remain intact. In retrograde amnesia, memories before the event are lost, while new memories can still be made.

Test 2: Questions

1. As the leader of your nursing team, you are responsible for delegating activities to any newly employed registered nurses and nursing assistants. Which of the following principles of delegation is most appropriate?

    A. Delegate according to nurses' level of education
    B. Delegate according to state statutes
    C. Delegate according to the scope of practice of the American Nurses Association
    D. Delegate according to nurses' age

2. As the head of your nursing team, your attention has been drawn to a team nurse who allegedly has poor time-management skills. Which of the following interventions is most appropriate?

    A. Observe the nurse during an entire shift.
    B. Interview the nurse's patients and note their response.
    C. Assign specific tasks to the nurse and collect data on his performance.
    D. Ask colleagues their impressions about the nurse.

3. A 66-year-old female who was admitted for a fracture of the neck of the femur divulges her current financial status. She is worried that she may not be able to cover future health bills. Which of the following interventions is appropriate?

    A. Inform her about Medicare.
    B. Inform her about Medicaid.
    C. Inform her of low-cost nursing homes.
    D. Start a GoFundMe account on her behalf.

4. You are discharging a patient who was admitted with a unilateral steppage gait due to peroneal nerve injury. Which of the following specialists is most appropriate for this patient?

    A. An occupational therapist
    B. A physical therapist
    C. A podiatrist
    D. A chiropractor

5. You are discharging a 56-year-old male who was recently diagnosed with stage 2 Parkinson's disease. Which of the following specialists is unsuitable for multidisciplinary care?

    A. A psychologist
    B. A psychiatrist
    C. An occupational therapist
    D. A podiatrist

6. Your attention has been drawn to an event that led to the physical harm of a patient. Which of the following best describes the event?

    A. Adverse effect
    B. Sentinel event
    C. Root cause event
    D. Iatrogenic effect

7. You are part of the committee set up to determine the factors that led to an incidence of negligence in a health unit. What is this process called?

    A. Troubleshooting
    B. Root-cause analysis
    C. Brainstorming
    D. Quality control

8. A patient with metastatic prostate cancer has just had a colostomy for intestinal obstruction. Which of the following interventions is inappropriate for facilitating wound healing?

    A. Change dressings as indicated
    B. Use sitz baths
    C. Irrigate wound with salt-poor albumin
    D. Place in the side-lying position with the head elevated

9. A patient with uncontrolled type 2 diabetes mellitus has just been placed on intravenous insulin for optimal glucose control. Which of the following statements is not true?

    A. Opened vials of insulin can be stored at a temperature of 15°C for one month.
    B. Symptoms of hypoglycemia include tachycardia, sweating and headaches.
    C. Shots should be rotated over multiple anatomic sites.
    D. Injection of insulin in the same site over time will cause lipoatrophy.

10. A patient is being managed for a severe head injury following a fall from a height. Which of the following interventions for eliminating urine is most appropriate?

    A. A bedpan
    B. An adult diaper
    C. A urethral catheter
    D. A suprapubic catheter

11. A patient is being managed for generalized seizures caused by an intracranial mass. Which of the following interventions is inappropriate for his care and comfort?

    A. IV diazepam
    B. Physical restraint
    C. An oropharyngeal airway
    D. Turning the patient to the left lateral position

12. A 55-year-old man has just had an amputation of his right leg for severe crush injury and is suffering from depression as a result of the procedure. Which of the following interventions is most appropriate?

    A. Encourage the patient to be grateful for his other leg.
    B. Refer the patient to a psychiatrist.
    C. Start the patient on an antidepressant.
    D. Encourage early ambulation.

13. A patient who has a cast for a fracture of the humerus complains of intense pruritus under the cast. Which of the following interventions is inappropriate?

    A. Rub the skin around the edge of the cast with alcohol.
    B. Encourage the patient to avoid scratching the itch.
    C. Line the edges of the cast with waterproof tape.
    D. Use zinc oxide on the affected area.

14. Which of the following measures is inappropriate for a 45-year-old male who just had a scotch vast for a right humeral fracture?

    A. Prop the affected limb up with a pillow.
    B. Encourage flexion of the digits on the affected limb.
    C. Apply ice bags intermittently on the affected limb.
    D. Split the cast at least 72 hours after it was applied.

15. Which of the following organizations protects the health information of patients and how it is being used?

    A. HIPAA
    B. Code of ethics
    C. Informed consent
    D. State board of nursing

16. A patient who has just been diagnosed with local invasive breast cancer insists that her husband should not be informed of her condition. Which of the following aspects of HIPPA applies?

    A. Security rule
    B. Privacy rule
    C. Breach notification rule
    D. Omnibus final rule

17. A patient who has been asked to take part in a clinical research trial is protected by all of the following except:

    A. Code of ethics
    B. HIPAA
    C. Informed consent
    D. State board of nursing

18. A patient declines treatment for his inguinal hernia for personal and religious reasons. After educating the patient on the implications of his decision, the AG-ACNP decides to respect the patient's wishes. Which aspect of ethics is being demonstrated?

    A. Beneficence
    B. Nonmaleficence
    C. Justice
    D. Autonomy

19. An AG-ACNP who uses a physical restraint on a patient experiencing an acute psychotic episode has demonstrated which of the following?

    A. Maltreatment
    B. Negligence
    C. Assault
    D. Nonmaleficence

20. An AG-ACNP forgets to remove the tourniquet from the arm of a delirious patient after a venipuncture. Two hours later, the patient's arm is discovered to be swollen. This can be considered...

A. Negligence
B. Assault
C. Malpractice
D. Battery

21. An AG-ACNP who says to a patient, "If you do not let me give you this IV drug, I won't attend to you anymore," has just demonstrated which of the following?

A. Justice
B. Maleficence
C. Assault
D. Battery

22. You are researching the efficacy of ventilators for people with acute respiratory distress syndrome. Which of the following is not a primary source for collecting your data?

A. Diaries
B. Newspapers
C. Case files
D. Journal articles

23. You have been asked to produce information on evidence-based debridement of wounds using sterile larvae. Which of the following sources of data is appropriate?

A. Journal articles
B. Case notes
C. Diaries
D. Newspapers

24. You are conducting qualitative research on the factors that affect the delivery of health care to homeless patients. Which of the following statements is correct?

    A. Your research will require quantification of specific observed phenomena.
    B. Your research will require close-ended questions.
    C. You may attempt to describe the cause and effect between these factors and the quality of health care given to homeless patients.
    D. You may attempt to describe how nurses feel about health-care delivery to homeless patients.

25. Nurse T is conducting research that can improve his clinical effectiveness. This means that he is focused on which of the following?

    A. Studying the effective outcomes of his research
    B. Creating new principles of clinical management
    C. Improving his effectiveness in leading his team
    D. Using evidence-based practice in improving nursing care

26. A key aspect of clinical inquiry is promoting the use of evidence-based practice in clinical settings. Which of the following is not an example of evidence-based practice?

    A. Infection control
    B. Oxygen supplementation in patients with COPD
    C. Acupuncture for fibromyalgia
    D. Size 18-gauge needle for red blood cell transfusion

27. Which of the following is not a component of evidence-based practice?

    A. Research evidence
    B. Patient's preference
    C. Clinical expertise
    D. Expected outcomes

28. Nurse M is doing qualitative research on the use of CPAP on patients with obstructive sleep apnea. Which of the following is not a tool for data collection?

    A. Open-ended questions
    B. Unstructured interviews
    C. Semi-structured interviews
    D. Focus group questionnaires

29. Nurse J is a new AG-ACNP who is starting his rotations in the ICU. Part of his compensation package includes an occurrence-based malpractice insurance coverage. Which of the following statements is accurate regarding that insurance?

    A. Nurse J. will require additional coverage.
    B. It offers coverage when a claim is made.
    C. It offers coverage on an incident even after a claim is made when the policy is not in effect.
    D. It protects the provider.

30. You discharge a 55-year-old female who was admitted with left cerebral ischemic stroke and refer her to an inpatient physiotherapy center. What level of prevention is this?

    A. Primary
    B. Secondary
    C. Tertiary
    D. Quaternary

31. You discharge a 25-year-old female who was admitted for pelvic inflammatory disease. Which of the following is a primary level of prevention?

    A. Prophylactic doxycycline
    B. Intrauterine contraceptive
    C. Barrier contraceptive
    D. Spermicide

32. According to the American Nurses Association, which of these is not the role of the acute care nurse practitioner?

    A. Leader
    B. Clinician
    C. Consultant
    D. Collaborator

33. You discharge an 85-year-old female who was admitted for a fracture of the hip. Which of the following teaching methods is most appropriate?

    A. Text-based leaflets on body alignment and exercise
    B. Video-based content on body alignment and exercise
    C. A video on hip surgery
    D. Oral instruction on exercise and body alignment techniques

34. A 16-year-old female who is nervous about an emergency appendectomy requests an explanation of the procedure. Which of the following interventions is most appropriate?

    A. Give her a copy of a surgical handbook.
    B. Watch a YouTube video of an appendectomy with her.
    C. Use a flowchart and diagrams to explain the procedure to her.
    D. Request that the attending surgeon explain the procedure to her.

35. A newly diagnosed hypertensive who was admitted for MI is about to be discharged on warfarin. Which of the following statements confirms that the patient understands the implications of warfarin?

    A. "If I cut myself when shaving, I will bleed extensively."
    B. "I should stop all herbal remedies except ginger tea."
    C. "I shouldn't eat too much cabbage and kale."
    D. "I should compensate for a missed dose by taking extra doses."

36. Nurse M expects her patient from Cambodia to drink green tea, so she adds it to her menu without asking. Which of the following is being demonstrated?

    A. Cultural appropriation
    B. Cultural stereotyping
    C. Cultural competency
    D. Cultural imposition

37. Nurse P refuses to attend to a gay patient admitted for appendicitis because she does not believe in same-sex marriage. Which of the following is demonstrated?

    A. Prejudice
    B. Discrimination
    C. Racism
    D. Bias

38. Nurse U observes that her Muslim patient may need privacy for his prayers. Which of the following did Nurse U demonstrate?

    A. Cultural awareness
    B. Cultural competence
    C. Empathy
    D. Social awareness

39. Nurse H understands that her Jewish patient has a regulatory code of eating, so she allows his wife to bring his food from home. Which of the following is being demonstrated?

A. Cultural awareness
B. Cultural competence
C. Empathy
D. Liberalism

40. Which of the following best explains the high mortality rates among homeless patients?

A. Lack of formal education
B. Suboptimal access to health care
C. Drug abuse and intoxication
D. Exposure to air pollutants

41. H is a Mexican patient who was admitted to the ER with diabetic ketoacidosis. You are about to discharge her when she tells you that she has been consulting with holistic healers for a cure for her diabetes. Which of the following interventions is appropriate?

A. Say nothing to avoid conflicts with her cultural beliefs.
B. Educate her on the limitations of such treatment.
C. Collect a history of the drugs she is using to avoid herb-drug interactions.
D. Offer to visit the holistic healers she has talked to, to gather more information.

42. Which of the following patients is most at risk of developing type 2 diabetes mellitus?

A. A 75-year-old Russian
B. A 65-year-old Black American
C. A 35-year-old Hispanic American
D. A 45-year-old Native American

43. Which of the following is a clinician barrier in patients' non-adherence?

A. Cost of medication/treatment
B. Lack of empathy for the patient's condition
C. Insufficient instruction on treatment modalities
D. Cultural bias

44. Which of the following is a system barrier against patient adherence and compliance?

    A. Insufficient health insurance
    B. Cost of medical care
    C. Inefficient discharge and follow-up
    D. Bureaucracy and bottleneck

45. Which of the following is not a social factor that affects adherence among patients?

    A. The patient's economic status
    B. Sexual orientation
    C. Culture and ethnicity
    D. Family support

46. Which of the following is not a reason for obtaining a detailed list of complementary therapies from your patient?

    A. To rule out drug-herb interactions
    B. To educate the patient on the limitations of such therapies
    C. To assess the patient's sociocultural orientation
    D. To measure the rate of response to standard therapy

47. Which of the following responses is inappropriate for a patient who wishes to be discharged against medical advice?

    A. Give verbal instructions and referrals on follow-up
    B. Document the patient's request for discharge
    C. Explain the implications of such a decision to the patient
    D. Inform social services

48. According to West African culture, which of these gestures is offensive?

    A. Direct eye contact
    B. Crossing the legs when seated
    C. Using the left hand to provide prescription notes
    D. Using the patient's full name

49. Your patient is a 35-year-old Mexican woman who has just been diagnosed with diabetes mellitus. Which of the following interventions is most appropriate in helping her with weight loss?

A. Sign her up for a keto class
B. Place her on a 1,000 calorie/day diet
C. Encourage her to avoid all oily and high-calorie meals
D. Refer her to a dietician

50. A 24-year-old male presents to the ER with left shoulder pain. On examination, there is tenderness, which is exacerbated when the shoulder joint is abducted at 120 degrees and absent when the shoulder is abducted at 180 degrees. Which of the following diagnoses is most likely?

A. Anterior dislocation of the shoulder
B. Posterior dislocation of the shoulder
C. Rotator cuff tears
D. Inferior dislocation of the shoulder

51. Which of the following is not an example of distributive shock?

A. Severe sepsis from endotoxin poisoning
B. Severe spinal injury at T4
C. Opioid overdose
D. Impaired myocardial contractility

52. A homeless man presents to the ER with fever, sore throat and a thick white plaque on the dorsum of the tongue. Significant findings on examination include marked wasting. Which of the following diagnoses is most appropriate?

A. Candidiasis
B. Leukoplakia
C. Stomatitis
D. Oral squamous cell carcinoma

53. An 80-year-old female is admitted to the ER with fecal impaction. Significant findings on examination include a history of oral opioids for chronic back pain. Which of the following interventions is most appropriate?

A. Lactulose
B. Bisacodyl
C. Phosphate enema
D. Omeprazole

54. A patient is being managed for an upper motor neuron lesion. Significant findings on examination include brisk deep tendon reflexes of the knee. Which of the following is the correct innervation for the knee jerk reflex?

A. S1
B. L4
C. S2
D. L5

55. Which of the following is not an organic cause of failure to thrive?

A. Malabsorption syndrome
B. Increased energy requirements
C. Increased excretion
D. Impoverishment

56. A patient is admitted with weakness, fatigue and dizziness. Significant findings on examination include angular stomatitis, glossitis, pallor and papulovesicular rashes on the elbows and knees. A history of passage of bulky, oily and foul-smelling stools is obtained. Which of the following diagnoses is most appropriate?

A. Celiac disease
B. Inflammatory bowel disease
C. Colorectal cancer
D. Chronic gastroenteritis

57. A patient presents to the ER with cough, chest pain and hemoptysis. A history of travel to Asia is obtained. Significant findings on investigations include eosinophilia and pulmonary infiltrates on a chest X-ray. Which of the following interventions is most appropriate?

A. Metronidazole therapy
B. Albendazole therapy
C. Piperazine therapy
D. Artemether therapy

58. A 25-year-old homeless patient is admitted with headaches, sore throat, trismus and risus sardonicus. Which of the following principles of management is inappropriate?

A. Prevention of excess stimuli
B. Antitoxin to neutralize bound tetanospasmin
C. Immunize with antitoxid
D. Sedate with a benzodiazepine

59. In assessing a patient with fever of unknown origin, which of the following is most appropriate?

A. The nurse practitioner should repeat blood-work tests to detect insidious causes.
B. The nurse practitioner should rely on the diagnosis of previous clinicians.
C. The nurse practitioner should pay close attention to fever patterns for diagnosis.
D. A review of systems should include both nonspecific symptoms and system-specific symptoms.

60. A 50-year-old female presents to the ER with bloody discharge and ulceration around her left nipple. On examination, there is itching, excoriation and erythema. Which of the following diagnoses is most appropriate?

A. Paget's disease of the breast
B. Fibrocystic dysplasia
C. Eczema
D. Duct papilloma

61. A 51-year-old female with metastatic ovarian carcinoma presents to the ER with abdominal pain and vomiting. Significant findings on examination include vomiting and hyperactive bowel sounds. Which of the following interventions is most appropriate?

A. Intravenous morphine
B. Hyoscine bromide
C. Colostomy
D. Lactulose

62. A 45-year-old female presents to the ER with severe abdominal pain and fever. Significant findings on examination are BMI 27 kg/m2, temp 38°C, pain in the right hypochondrium and parity of five children. Which of the following diagnoses is most likely?

A. Cholecystitis
B. Hepatitis A
C. Ovarian torsion
D. Ectopic pregnancy

63. A patient who is being managed for acute myeloblastic leukemia complains of fever, chills and rigors. Hematologic tests are as follows:

RBC: 10 g/dL; platelets: 15,000/uL; WBC: 400/uL. The temperature on examination is 38°C. Which of the following interventions is inappropriate?

A. Emergency chest X-ray
B. Examination for possible abscesses
C. IV ceftazidime
D. Digital rectal examination

64. A patient on radiation therapy complains of anorexia and pain in the buccal mucosa. Significant findings on examination include redness and swelling of the mucosa of the mouth. Which of the following interventions is inappropriate?

A. Mouth rinses with 2% viscous lidocaine before meals
B. Use of a nasogastric tube
C. Oral nystatin suspension
D. Avoid citrus juice

65. A patient with aplastic anemia complains of constipation from the chronic use of opioids. Which of the following interventions is inappropriate?

    A. Bisacodyl
    B. Lactulose
    C. Milk of magnesia
    D. Enema

66. A patient who is suffering from opioid withdrawal is unlikely to have which of these symptoms?

    A. Diaphoresis
    B. Mydriasis
    C. Hypertension
    D. Miosis

67. Which of the following statements is false in differentiating delirium from dementia?

    A. Delirium affects attention, while dementia affects memory.
    B. Delirium is sudden in onset, while dementia is insidious.
    C. Delirium is usually reversible, while dementia is not.
    D. The level of consciousness in delirium is more impaired than that in dementia.

68. A patient diagnosed with bipolar disorder was recently placed on lithium. Which of the following is not a risk factor for lithium toxicity?

    A. Impaired renal function
    B. Advanced age
    C. Use of diuretics
    D. Hypothyroidism

69. A 19-year-old female has just been placed on sertraline for severe depression. Which of the following information is necessary for the patient?

    A. A risk of toxicity, which includes malignant hyperthermia
    B. A risk of suicidal ideas and attempts
    C. A risk of nephrotoxicity
    D. A risk of hypertensive crises

70. A hypertensive patient who just had a recent MI has been recently diagnosed with depression. Which of the following antidepressants is suitable for this patient?

   A. Lofepramine
   B. Sertraline
   C. Citalopram
   D. Fluoxetine

71. A patient is currently being managed for raised intracranial hypertension secondary to an intracranial tumor. Which of the following interventions is inappropriate?

   A. Elevating the head of the bed to 30 degrees
   B. Maintain serum osmolality to 295 to 320 mOsm/kg
   C. Nasotracheal intubation
   D. Sedation

72. A patient is given IV mannitol for raised ICP. Which of the following statements is false regarding the treatment?

   A. Mannitol is an osmotic diuretic.
   B. Mannitol rapidly expands intravascular volume; therefore IV Lasix is required.
   C. Mannitol is given over 45 minutes.
   D. Prolonged mannitol use can cause hypernatremia.

73. A 25-year-old male is admitted for bacterial meningitis. Which of the following signs is unlikely to be found in this patient?

   A. Involuntary flexion of the hips when there is a passive flexion of the neck
   B. Incomplete extension of the knee when the thigh is flexed at 90 degrees to the trunk
   C. Hyperemic swollen disk
   D. Global hypertonia

74. The AG-ACNP is performing a lumbar puncture on a patient with suspected bacterial meningitis. Which of the following steps is incorrect?

   A. Place the patient in the left lateral decubitus position.
   B. Swab the skin with povidone-iodine and alcohol.
   C. Palpate for the anterior superior iliac spine, which connects the two iliac crests across the L4 spinous process.
   D. Aim the needle rostrally toward the patient's umbilicus.

75. A patient just had a lumbar puncture for suspected bacterial meningitis. Which of the following parameters is unlikely on CSF analysis?

    A. A preponderance of lymphocytes
    B. Elevated CSF protein
    C. Turbid CSF
    D. CSF glucose <50% of blood glucose

76. The following is the CSF analysis result of a patient who is being managed in the ER for headaches, fever and projectile vomiting. Opening pressure 210 mmH20, WBC 3/muL, glucose 5 mmol/L, protein 40 mg/dL. Which of the following diagnoses is most appropriate?

    A. Bacterial meningitis
    B. Viral meningitis
    C. Cerebral hemorrhage
    D. Idiopathic intracranial hypertension

77. A patient experiences a loss of consciousness that lasts for about 30 seconds with an associated fluttering of the eyelids and anterograde amnesia. There is no loss of axial muscle tone, convulsions or postal ictal incontinence. What type of seizure disorder is this?

    A. Focal impaired awareness seizures
    B. Focal aware seizures
    C. Absence seizures
    D. Epilepsia partialis continua

78. A patient recently diagnosed with a seizure disorder is to be placed on antiseizure drugs. Which of the following is not a risk for relapse?

    A. A seizure disorder that began from childhood
    B. Focal onset seizures
    C. Structural brain lesions
    D. General onset seizures

79. A patient is admitted with flaccid weakness of the arms and lower limbs. There is a history of burning sensation and weakness occurring in the lower limbs that later progressed to the arms. On examination, there is a loss of deep tendon reflex. Which of the following diagnoses is most likely?

A. ALS
B. PLS
C. Guillain-Barré syndrome
D. Poliomyelitis

80. A patient has a gait that makes him lift his left foot higher than normal to prevent dragging the affected foot on the floor. Which of the following diagnoses is most likely?

A. Posterior circulation stroke
B. Foot drop
C. Muscular dystrophy
D. Huntington's disease

81. A patient walks into the ER with his right arm flexed, adducted and internally rotated. His right leg is extended with plantar flexion of the foot and toes. Which of the following diagnoses is most appropriate?

A. Ischemic stroke
B. Cerebral palsy
C. Foot drop
D. Muscular dystrophy

82. A patient walks into the ER dragging both of his legs and scraping his toes. Which of the following diagnoses is most appropriate?

A. Cerebral palsy
B. Foot drop
C. ALS
D. Guillain-Barré

83. A patient presents to the ER with a waddling gait. Which of the following diagnoses is most appropriate?

A. Muscular dystrophy
B. Stroke
C. Peroneal nerve palsy
D. Sciatica

84. A 22-year-old female, a known seizure disorder patient, is admitted with widespread blisters on the trunk, arms, legs and mucocutaneous surfaces. Significant findings on examination are widespread slough covering about 5 percent of the body's surface area. Which of the following diagnoses is most appropriate?

    A. Bullous pemphigoid
    B. Steven Johnson syndrome
    C. Toxic epidermal necrolysis
    D. Exfoliative erythredema

85. A 25-year-old female presents with intense itching of both hands. Significant findings on examination include vesicles and erythema, which are worse on the left wrist. Which of the following diagnoses is most appropriate?

    A. Seborrheic dermatitis
    B. Irritant dermatitis
    C. Allergic contact dermatitis
    D. Atopic dermatitis

86. A 34-year-old male is admitted with intense itching and restlessness. Important findings on examination include yellowing and scaling of the trunk and extremities, particularly the palms and soles. Red follicular papules that merge into scaling plaques are noticed on the palms and soles. Which of the following diagnoses is most likely?

    A. Pityriasis rosea
    B. Psoriasis
    C. Pityriasis rubra pilaris
    D. Lichen planus

87. Which of the following best describes stage 2 kidney disease?

    A. eGFR 30 to 59
    B. eGFR 60 to 89
    C. eGFR 15 to 29
    D. eGFR 30 to 49

88. A patient is having a contrast CT angiography of the coronary arteries. Which of the following is not a risk factor for contrast nephrotoxicity?

    A. Multiple myeloma
    B. Diabetes mellitus
    C. Nonionic contrast agents
    D. Hyperosmolar contrast agents

89. Which of the following parameters is used to diagnose contrast nephropathy in a patient who has just had a contrast CT of the carotid arteries?

    A. Serum urea
    B. Serum creatinine
    C. Serum BUN
    D. Serum potassium

90. A patient is admitted to the ER with dizziness, abdominal and joint pain and fatigue. Significant findings include BP 150/100 mmHg, flank pain, dysuria and hematuria. There is a history of chronic use of aspirin for joint pain. Which of the following diagnoses is most accurate?

    A. Focal segmental glomerulosclerosis
    B. Analgesic nephropathy
    C. SLE
    D. Hypertensive kidney disease

91. A 55-year-old male is admitted to the ER with an inability to void urine and suprapubic pain. A significant finding on examination is a palpable bladder. DRE reveals an enlarged prostate with stony, hard nodules that extend to the seminal vesicles. Which of the following diagnoses is appropriate?

    A. Benign prostatic hyperplasia
    B. Prostatic cancer
    C. Prostatitis
    D. Prostate calculi

92. Which of the following is not a cause of hyperkalemia?

    A. Paralytic ileus
    B. Hypoaldosteronism
    C. ACEIs
    D. Diabetes mellitus

93. A patient being managed for ESRD presents with muscle weakness and tingling sensation in the upper and lower limbs. Biochemical results are as follows: urea, 9 mmol/L; creatinine, 400 umol/L; K, 6.5 mmol/L. ECG findings include tall T waves and shortened QRS interval. Which of the following interventions is expedient?

    A. Hemodialysis
    B. IV calcium gluconate
    C. Nebulized salbutamol
    D. Insulin dextrose infusion

94. Which of the following is not a cause of upper GI bleeding?

    A. Mallory Weiss tear
    B. Esophageal varices
    C. Peptic ulcer disease
    D. Anorectal fissure

95. Which of the following is not a feature of chronic liver disease?

    A. Dupuytren's contracture
    B. Testicular atrophy
    C. Spider nevi
    D. Spoon-shaped nails

96. A 57-year-old male presents to the ER with complaints of fatigue, nausea, vomiting and palpitations. Physical examination reveals hepatomegaly, ascites, wasting and a palpable mass in the left supraclavicular space. Which of the following diagnoses is most likely?

    A. Gastric carcinoma
    B. Colorectal carcinoma
    C. Peptic ulcer disease
    D. Atrophic gastritis

97. Which of the following is not a typical feature of right colon cancer?

    A. Bloating
    B. Fatigue
    C. Hematemesis
    D. Syncope

98. A 55-year-old male presents to the ER with fatigue, dizziness and abdominal pain. On examination, he is icteric and febrile (38°C)and has tender hepatomegaly. A hepatic bruit is heard on auscultation. Which of the following diagnoses is most unlikely?

    A. Cirrhosis
    B. Alcoholic hepatitis
    C. Hepatic steatosis
    D. Hepatoma

99. A patient has just been diagnosed with alcoholic hepatitis secondary to alcoholic liver disease. Which of the following statements is false pertaining to the patient's condition?

    A. Alcohol abstinence is the main treatment.
    B. Opioids are useful for advanced cases of alcoholic liver disease.
    C. Diazepams are useful for alcohol withdrawal symptoms.
    D. Enteral feeding may be needed for severe cases of alcoholic liver disease.

100. A patient is to receive 6 L of whole blood for a massive hemorrhage. Which of the following principles is not useful?

    A. Use of IV calcium gluconate
    B. Use of heated blankets and warmers
    C. Use of intravenous Lasix
    D. Use of intravenous potassium

101. You are transfusing two units of RBCs to a patient involved in a traffic accident. Which of the following is not an early complication of RBC transfusion?

    A. Allergic reaction
    B. Non-febrile hemolytic reaction
    C. Post-transfusion purpura
    D. Chill-rigor reactions

102. Which of the following best describes type 1 hypersensitivity reactions?

    A. They are mediated by IgG
    B. They are also called delayed hypersensitivity reaction
    C. Examples include urticaria
    D. Examples include nephrotic syndrome

103. Autoimmune hemolytic anemia is an example of which hypersensitivity reaction?

    A. Type I
    B. Type II
    C. Type III
    D. Type IV

104. A 24-year-old presents to the hospital with altered consciousness, diarrhea and shortness of breath following a sushi meal at an upscale restaurant. Significant findings on examination include PR 100 bpm, BP 100/60 mmHg and RR 45 cpm. On examination, there are raised reddish welts on the arms, trunk and legs. Which of the following interventions is inappropriate?

    A. Supplemental oxygen
    B. Epinephrine
    C. Nebulized salbutamol
    D. IV atenolol

105. Which of the following is not an example of a drug hypersensitivity reaction?

    A. Serum sickness
    B. Drug-induced hemolytic anemia
    C. SLE-like syndrome
    D. Peripheral neuropathy

106. A 45-year-old female is rushed to the ER with altered consciousness and severe abdominal pain. Significant findings on examination include temp 38°C, PR 120 bpm, BP 100/60 mmHg and diffused hyperpigmentation on her elbows, areolas and the mucosal membranes of the mouth. Which of the following diagnoses is most appropriate?

    A. Bronchogenic Ca
    B. Hemochromatosis
    C. Addison's disease
    D. Cushing syndrome

107. Which of the following investigations is inappropriate for a patient with Cushing's disease?

   A. Synacthen test
   B. Dexamethasone suppression test
   C. Urinary free cortisol measurement
   D. ACTH stimulation test

108. Which of the following best describes the pathophysiology of Cushing's disease?

   A. Excess production of Hemoglobin
   B. Excess secretion of ACTH from a non-pituitary tumor
   C. Administration of corticosteroid
   D. Secreting adrenal carcinoma

109. A known type 2 diabetic is rushed to the ER with altered consciousness, nausea and vomiting. Investigations reveal RBS 300 mg/dL, serum ketone 4 mmol/L, HCO3 18 mmol/L. Which of the following management principles is inappropriate?

   A. Rehydration with 0.9% normal saline
   B. Insulin therapy when potassium is 3 mmol/L
   C. Potassium replacement therapy
   D. IV mannitol for cerebral edema

110. Which of the following is not a feature of alcoholic ketoacidosis?

   A. Ketonemia
   B. High anion gap metabolic acidosis
   C. Hyperglycemia
   D. Hypokalemia

111. Which of the following is false concerning nephrogenic diabetes insipidus?

   A. There is an insufficient secretion of vasopressin.
   B. There is an inability to concentrate urine in the presence of vasopressin.
   C. Lithium can be a cause.
   D. Water deprivation test is diagnostic.

112. A 37-year-old female is rushed to the ER with difficulty breathing, restlessness and chest pain. Significant findings on examination include distension of the neck veins, peripheral edema and peripheral cyanosis that persists even after oxygen supplementation. An emergency chest X-ray reveals diffused infiltrate in the lung, cardiomegaly and a wide vascular pedicle. Which of the following best explains the pathophysiology of the patient's condition?

    A. Lung collapse and surfactant dysfunction
    B. Right to left shunting of blood
    C. Elevated alveolar hydrostatic pressure
    D. Inflammatory exudates in the lung parenchyma

113. Patient Y is a 34-year-old male who was admitted to the ER with difficulty breathing and altered consciousness. Significant findings on examination include PR 100 bpm, RR 44 cpm, temp 39°C and SPO2 86% even with supplemental oxygen. A chest examination reveals hyporesonant notes and bronchial breath sounds on the left hemithorax. Which of the following interventions is most appropriate?

    A. Thoracentesis
    B. Antipyretic treatment
    C. Mechanical ventilation
    D. Emergency chest X-ray

114. Patient G has just been placed on a mechanical ventilator for acute respiratory distress syndrome. Which of the following principles is inappropriate in improving respiratory function?

    A. Administering opioids to reduce anxiety
    B. Suctioning to reduce the risk of blockage
    C. Positioning the patient in the high Fowler's position as tolerated
    D. Using nasal prongs for improved oxygen delivery

115. A patient on a mechanical ventilator suddenly develops shortness of breath and chest pain. Significant findings on chest examination include RR 34 cpm, tracheal is central, absent tactile fremitus, decreased breath sounds and hyperresonant percussion notes on the right hemithorax. Which of the following diagnoses is most appropriate?

    A. Cardiac tamponade
    B. Hemothorax
    C. Pneumothorax
    D. ARD

116. A patient on mechanical ventilation suddenly develops substernal chest pain that increases in severity. A chest examination reveals a positive Hamman's sign. Which of the following is most likely to be seen on a chest X-ray?

    A. Subcutaneous emphysema
    B. Blunted costophrenic angle
    C. Kerley B lines
    D. Unfolding of the aorta

117. A patient on mechanical ventilation complains of sudden onset of breathlessness, dizziness and restlessness. On examination, the patient is tachypneic and tachycardic. Blood pressure is 90/60 mmHg, and there are visible distended external jugular veins. On chest examination, the trachea is deviated to the right, and there are hyperresonant sounds in the left hemithorax. Which of the following interventions is most appropriate?

    A. Emergency chest X-ray
    B. Emergency thoracocentesis
    C. Emergency thoracotomy
    D. Emergency tracheostomy

118. A 56-year-old patient is admitted to the ER with shortness of breath, stridor and swelling of the face and lips. Significant findings on examination include tachypnea, tachycardia and added breath sounds. SP02 in atmospheric oxygen is 86%. Which of the following interventions is appropriate?

    A. Give supplemental oxygen.
    B. Secure an airway with an endotracheal tube.
    C. Give IV prednisolone.
    D. Give IV antihistamine.

119. A tall and thin 18-year-old male presents to the ER with complaints of sudden chest pain and breathlessness. He is anxious and becomes increasingly breathless when he cries. Which of the following is the most appropriate investigation?

    A. ECG
    B. Echocardiography
    C. Chest X-ray
    D. CT pulmonary angiography

120. A construction foreman presents to the ER with an inability to move his right arm following a fall. A diagnosis of fracture of the right humerus is made. During the history, the patient complains of morning headaches, hypersomnolence, fatigue and impaired concentration. Which of the following diagnoses is most appropriate?

   A. Substance abuse disorder
   B. Vitamin B deficiency
   C. Migraine
   D. Obstructive sleep apnea

121. You are managing a patient with pulmonary edema secondary to left ventricular heart failure. The patient is on supplemental oxygen via nasal prongs. However, you notice that the patient gasps and snores intermittently when asleep. A history of morning headaches, fatigue and impaired concentration is obtained from the patient. Which of the following investigations is appropriate?

   A. Brain MRI
   B. Bronchoscopy
   C. Sleep studies
   D. Chest X-ray

122. A 45-year-old male presents to the ER with complaints of shortness of breath, non-productive cough and chest pain. Significant findings on chest examination include deviation of the trachea to the right and hyporesonant percussion notes on the left hemithorax. Vital signs include BP 120/80 mmHg, PR 82b pm, RR 35 cpm. A history of 20 years is obtained. On thoracostomy, a copious amount of serosanguinous fluid is drained. Which of the following diagnoses is most appropriate?

   A. Pulmonary tuberculosis
   B. COPD
   C. Bronchogenic CA
   D. Massive hemothorax

123. Which of the following is not a pathologic feature of emphysema?

   A. Loss of elastic recoil
   B. Lung hyperinflation
   C. Radial airway traction
   D. Mucus plugs

124. Patient R is a 45-year-old male being managed for emphysema. He presents to the ER with exacerbated symptoms of shortness of breath and fatigue. On examination, he has distended jugular veins, pedal edema and a left parasternal systolic lift. Which of the following diagnoses is most appropriate?

    A. Pulmonary hypertension
    B. Cor pulmonale
    C. Right ventricular failure
    D. Pulmonary carcinoma

125. Which of the following is false about the principles of PCI?

    A. Anticoagulation therapy is used to reduce the risk of thrombosis.
    B. Calcium channel blockers are used to reduce vasospasms.
    C. It is indicated for patients with less than 50% occlusion.
    D. It may be done without stent insertion.

126. Which of the following patients will benefit from a stress test?

    A. A 58-year-old man with hypercholesterolemia and dyspnea on exertion
    B. A 55-year-old woman with recent myocardial infarction
    C. A 54-year-old man with symptomatic bundle branch block
    D. A 63-year-old man with decompensated heart failure

127. A 25-year-old male presents to the ER with cyanosis, burning pain and needle-like sensations on both fingers. There is a history of exposure to cold. Which of the following is the most likely diagnosis?

    A. Secondary Reynaud's syndrome
    B. Frostbite
    C. Primary Reynaud's syndrome
    D. Diabetic neuropathy

128. Which of the following is not a cause of distributive shock?

    A. Severe sepsis
    B. Urticaria
    C. Congestive heart failure
    D. Severe spinal injury

129. Which of the following is the most appropriate immediate intervention for a patient who has been diagnosed with atrial fibrillation?

A. Increased atrioventricular conduction
B. Thrombolytics therapy
C. Anxiolytic therapy
D. Increased coronary artery perfusion

130. Which of the following is the most prominent ECG finding in a patient with hyperkalemia?

A. Tall tented T waves
B. ST-segment elevation
C. Shortened PR segment
D. Tall P waves

131. Which electrolyte imbalance presents with widespread ST segments depression and inversion of the T waves?

A. Hyperkalemia
B. Hypercalcemia
C. Hypokalemia
D. Hypocalcemia

132. Which of the following abnormalities presents with an initial QRS deflection, shortened PR interval and prolonged QRS duration?

A. Atrial fibrillation
B. Torsades de Pointes
C. Ventricular tachycardia
D. Wolff-Parkinson-White syndrome

133. In interpreting an ECG strip, which of the following statements is false?

A. The P wave indicates depolarization of the atria.
B. The T wave indicates ventricular diastole.
C. The QRS complex indicates ventricular systole.
D. The T wave lasts for approximately 270 ms.

134. A 54-year-old male is admitted to the ER with symptoms of crushing chest pain, diaphoresis and nausea. Significant findings include BP 140/90 mmHg, PR 100 bpm, RR 34 cpm, BMI 25 kg/m2. Significant findings on ECG include ST-segment elevation in leads V1, V3, V5 and V6. What part of the patient's heart is being affected?

A. The posterior wall
B. The interior wall
C. The anterior wall
D. The lateral wall

135. Patient M is a 25-year-old varsity athlete being managed for hypertrophic cardiomyopathy. Which of the following statements is incorrect pertaining to the patient's condition?

A. Pharmacological intervention is with beta-blockers, calcium channel blockers and diuretics.
B. Syncope increases the risk for sudden death.
C. Blood pressure and heart rate are usually normal.
D. A systolic ejection murmur is heard in the obstructive type.

136. Patient H is being managed for systolic heart failure caused by hypertensive heart disease. He has just been placed on spironolactone for better blood pressure control. Which of the following principles of spironolactone therapy is false?

A. All potassium supplements should be stopped.
B. Serum potassium and creatinine analysis should be done biweekly for the first four to six weeks.
C. Spironolactone is an ACE inhibitor and a potassium-sparing diuretic.
D. Spironolactone therapy should be stopped if serum potassium is greater than 5.5 mEq.

137. A 57-year-old patient being managed for systolic heart failure is placed on furosemide. Which of the following is incorrect about the function of furosemide?

A. It reduces cardiac preload.
B. It is a potassium-sparing diuretic.
C. Hypovolemia is a serious complication of its use.
D. It is a loop diuretic.

138. Which of the following patients will benefit from digoxin therapy?

    A. A 53-year-old man with diastolic heart failure
    B. A 55-year-old woman with chronic atrial arrhythmia
    C. A 45-year-old hypertensive woman with acute pulmonary edema
    D. A 45-year-old hypertensive with congestive heart failure

139. Patient M is a newly diagnosed hypertensive. He has no complaints of dyspnea on exertion or edema. He has just been placed on amlodipine. Which of the following statements is correct pertaining to treatment?

    A. Stop all potassium-containing supplements.
    B. A dry cough is a side effect of amlodipine.
    C. Pedal edema is a side effect of amlodipine.
    D. Amlodipine should be taken when experiencing angina.

140. Patient M is a 34-year-old professional basketball player recently diagnosed with hypertrophic cardiomyopathy. Which of the following pharmacological interventions is inappropriate?

    A. Amiodarone
    B. Amlodipine
    C. Atenolol
    D. Digoxin

141. Patient Z is a 68-year-old hypertensive patient. He complains that he can't see properly and that his vision is blurry. After doing some tests, you notice ventricular tachycardia and fibrillation as symptoms. Which of the following is likely the diagnosis?

    A. Digoxin toxicity.
    B. Liver disease.
    C. Eye infection.
    D. Eye deterioration.

142. A 35-year-old man presents to the ER with dyspnea, diaphoresis, restlessness and chest pain. On examination, his blood pressure is 140/100 mmHg, PR is 120 bpm and RR is 45 cpm. Oxygen saturation is 80% in room oxygen. On respiratory examination, his trachea is central, with bilateral basal crepitations on both lungs. An emergency chest X-ray shows cephalization of the pulmonary vessels and Kerley B lines. After administering oxygen, what is the most appropriate line of action?

A. Thoracocentesis
B. Intravenous hydrocortisone
C. Intravenous furosemide
D. Nebulized salbutamol

143. J is a 26-year-old patient who presents to the ER with complaints of breathlessness, chest pain and cough. On examination, he is toxic, febrile and dyspneic. His oxygen saturation is 85% in room oxygen. Respiratory examination reveals hyporesonant sounds on the left hemithorax and bronchial breath sounds. Which of the following should be the first-line response?

A. Administration of IV antipyretics
B. Pleural aspiration
C. Emergency chest X-ray
D. Administration of oxygen

144. M is a 65-year-old patient who presents to the ER with complaints of crushing precordial pain, headaches and dizziness. On examination, BP is 150/100 mmHg, PR is 100 bpm, RR is 40 cpm, oxygen saturation at room temperature is 85%, breath sounds are vesicular. Which of the following initial responses is appropriate?

A. Give sublingual nitroglycerin.
B. Do an emergency ECG.
C. Administer IV morphine.
D. Give supplemental oxygen.

145. Patient H is a 55-year-old hypertensive with systolic heart failure. He is placed on oral digoxin, furosemide and lisinopril. He complains of green-yellow halos around lights. Which of the following responses is appropriate?

A. Refer the patient to an ophthalmologist for macula examination.
B. Stop digoxin.
C. Reduce furosemide dose by half.
D. Stop lisinopril.

146. Patient T is an 80-year-old male with a history of fainting spells. He presents to the ER following a gardening activity with his grandchildren. On examination, BP is 120/80 mmHg and PR is 72 bpm, full volume and regular. CVS examination reveals a systolic murmur. Which of the following investigations is diagnostic of his condition?

A. Chest X-ray
B. ECG
C. Echocardiography
D. 24-hour BP monitoring

147. A 54-year-old female presents to the ER with altered consciousness, confusion and agitation. Which of the following is not a component of the mini-mental state examination?

A. Orientation
B. Registration
C. Recall
D. Imagination

148. Which of the following instructions should be given to the patient from question 147 to assess her language skills?

A. What time of the day is it?
B. Take this paper, fold it in two and give it to me.
C. Can you draw a shape for me?
D. Subtract 5 from 100.

149. You take the blood pressure of a patient who is admitted with suspected heart failure. Which of the following principles of blood pressure measurement is incorrect?

A. A small cuff can create a falsely elevated reading.
B. Automated blood pressure methods use the oscillometric principle.
C. The auscultatory method involves listening to arterial sounds.
D. There are six Korotkoff sounds.

150. You perform a cardiovascular examination on a patient with hypertensive heart disease. Which of the following principles of cardiovascular examination is incorrect?

A. Auscultation of the heart
B. Palpation for heart sounds and murmurs
C. Inspection of jugular venous pressure
D. Percussion for cardiac size

Test 2: Answers and Explanations

1. (B) Delegate according to the state statutes.

This is the most objective criterion because state statutes give the legal job description of the different classes of nurses, including their limitations. Option A is incorrect because qualified nurses are expected to have the same standard of education. Option C is incorrect because the American Nurses Association does not have the scope of practice. Option D is discriminatory.

2. (C) Assign specific tasks to the nurse and collect data on his performance.

This is the most objective way to assess the nurse's time-management skills. The other options are subjective and liable to bias. Also, the other options do not give you first-hand knowledge of the nurse's skills and abilities.

3. (A) Inform her about Medicare.

This woman is qualified for Medicare, a health insurance program provided by the federal government. Option B is incorrect because it is hard to say if the patient has a low income. Option C is incorrect because nursing homes are for people who are unable to take care of themselves. Option D may be a breach of the patient's confidentiality.

4. (B) Physical therapist.

This patient has a foot drop caused by a peroneal nerve injury. Physical therapists provide interventions for patients with functional impairment in gait, mobility, balance, coordination, strength and range of motion. They do so by assessing the patient's range of function and providing exercises and additive aids.

5. (D) Podiatrist.

Podiatrists are specialists who manage disorders of the foot. Although they may collaborate with a physiotherapist in managing patients with mobility, gait and coordination disorders, podiatrists are unsuitable for this patient who requires multidisciplinary care. Specialists who are appropriate for this patient include psychiatrists, psychologists, dieticians, occupational therapists, neurologists and others.

6. (B) Sentinel event.

According to the Joint Commission, a sentinel event is an event in a health setting that leads to the death or serious physical and/or psychological harm of a patient. This event is not related to the natural progression of a disease.

7. (B) Root-cause analysis.

Root-cause analysis is done to identify the causes of problems in the health-care team. The overall aim of root-cause analysis is not to assign blame but to discover the factors that made it feasible for the problems to occur.

8. (C) Irrigate the wound with salt-poor albumin.

This intervention is inappropriate because the wound should be irrigated with normal saline, hydrogen peroxide or an antibiotic solution.

9. (C) Shots should be rotated over multiple anatomic sites.

This statement is false because skin absorption is consistent when insulin is injected in the same anatomical site. The American Diabetic Association advises that insulin be administered in the subcutaneous tissue of the abdomen.

10. (C) A urethral catheter.

A urethral catheter is most appropriate in this patient because acute management involves strict input and monitoring of fluids. Although an adult diaper can reduce the risk of urinary tract infections, it is quite difficult to measure the fluid output with an adult diaper.

11. (B) Physical restraint.

This intervention is inappropriate because IV sedatives are enough for controlling the seizures. Thereafter, antiseizure drugs can be started. A physical restraint like metallic cuffs is inappropriate unless the patient has status epilepticus and is at risk of causing injury to himself and others.

12. (B) Refer the patient to the psychiatrist.

This patient has clinical depression, which may become chronic. It is appropriate to refer him to the psychiatrist for expert management. Although early ambulation has its physical and psychological benefits, it may not be useful in helping this patient cope with depression.

13. (D) Use zinc oxide on the affected area.

This statement is inappropriate because creams and oils can seal the edges of the cast, preventing the skin underneath from breathing. Powders can also accumulate inside the cast and further irritate the skin. Rubbing alcohol is preferable because it dries up moisture on the skin.

14. (D) Split the cast at least 72 hours after it was applied.

This procedure is inappropriate because splitting/bivalving the cast should be done only when indicated. Bivalving is only an emergency procedure when there is a suspicion of compartment syndrome to relieve restriction and improve blood flow to the affected limb.

15. (A) HIPAA.

The Health Insurance Portability and Accountability Act (HIPAA) regulates the use and circulation of patients' health information. This involves privacy rules, as well as the breach notification rule, unique identifiers rule, security transaction rule, omnibus final rule and the HITECH Act.

16. (B) Privacy rule.

The privacy rule gives the patient a right to how her health information is used. This rule ensures that the patient's health information is kept in the utmost confidence and used only to provide the utmost health care.

17. (D) State board of nursing.

The state board of nursing is primarily responsible for setting and updating the standards of nursing care and its scope of practice and issuing licenses to qualified candidates.

18. (D) Autonomy.

In autonomy, the health-care provider respects the fact that the patient has the full right and freedom to make decisions about his health and how it is managed without any interference from second parties.

19. (D) Nonmaleficence.

The principle of nonmaleficence ensures that intentional harm is not done to others. In this case, the patient suffering from an acute psychotic episode is at risk of not only harming himself but others around him.

20. (A) Negligence.

Negligence in nursing is the inability to give a patient due attention. This may cause irresponsible actions and/or omission on the part of the nurse.

21. (C) Assault.

In nursing, assault is the intentional act of making someone afraid that harm might befall them. . In assault, the perpetrator does not have to cause harm to be guilty. Threats alone can constitute assault.

22. (D) Journal articles.

A primary source of data contains raw information that has not yet been classified or analyzed. They contain only the description and quantification of data. Primary sources of data include first-hand experience, diary entries, newspapers, audio and video recordings, photographs, case notes and other legal documents.

23. (A) Journal articles.

Evidence-based information must be obtained from analyzed data, not descriptive data in its raw form. Data that is obtained from journal entries is not only objective but has already been analyzed for interpretation and application.

24. (D) You may attempt to describe how nurses feel about health-care delivery to homeless patients.

Qualitative research is used to explore and describe phenomena. This method of research uses flexible study designs, open-ended questions and unstructured and semi-structured methods to categorize information and data.

25. (D) Using evidence-based practice in improving nursing care.

Clinical effectiveness is focused on improving the delivery of health care by using evidence-based practices. The outcomes of these practices are then evaluated and documented for future reference.

26. (C) Acupuncture for fibromyalgia.

Although acupuncture is regarded as an alternative therapy for chronic pain, there is not enough scientific evidence to make acupuncture a standardized and evidence-based practice.

27. (D) Expected outcomes.

The major components of evidence-based practices include researching the best external evidence, which must be clinically relevant and methodologically sound, respecting the patient's preferences and the clinical expertise of the nurse practitioner. Other minor components include the patient's clinical state, the clinical setting and circumstances that affect the feasibility of the practice.

28. (D) Focus group questionnaires.

This is not a tool for data collection. The methods used for collecting data for qualitative research include flexible study designs, open-ended questions, unstructured and semi-structured interviews and focus groups.

29. (C) It offers coverage on an incident even after a claim is made when the policy is not in effect.

Occurrence-based malpractice insurance protects against any incident that occurred when the policy was valid, even after a claim is made when the policy is no longer valid.

30. (C) Tertiary.

In the tertiary level of prevention, the patient is managed for complications arising from the progression of the disease. The purpose of the tertiary level of prevention is to improve the quality of living.

31. (C) Barrier contraceptive.

Primary prevention aims to prevent the occurrence of disease by reducing the risk of contracting illnesses. In this patient, the use of barrier contraceptives will reduce the risk of contracting a sexually transmitted infection.

32. (A) Leader.

According to the American Nurses Association, the five roles outlined for the acute care nurse practitioner include clinician, consultant, collaborator, consultant and educator.

33. (D) Oral instruction on exercise and body alignment techniques.

This teaching method is most appropriate for this elderly patient because you can assess her recall and understanding of what was said.

34. (B) Watch a YouTube video of an appendectomy with her.

This method is most appropriate because teenagers are curious and open to information. A YouTube video is most likely to answer all her questions because it is real and original. Watching the video with the patient allows her to ask questions and get comfortable about the surgery.

35. (C) "I shouldn't eat too much cabbage and kale."

Patients on warfarin are advised not to eat an excess of vitamin K-rich foods like kale, cabbage, brussels sprouts, green tea and cauliflower. These vegetables can counteract the effect of the anticoagulant and cause clotting. Option A is incorrect because although bleeding may occur during shaving, this occurrence is not normal and should be reported. Option B is incorrect because ginger is a natural anticoagulant that can thin the blood even further and cause bleeding. Option C is incorrect because warfarin has a narrow therapeutic index.

36. (B) Cultural stereotyping.

This occurs when someone expects another person to act in a certain way because of their ethnicity and cultural background.

37. (B) Discrimination.

Discrimination occurs when differential treatment is given to someone who is perceived to be lesser in status of sex, race, religion, socioeconomic power and age.

38. (A) Cultural awareness.

Cultural awareness occurs when someone recognizes and appreciates the values that characterize different cultures and their beliefs and value systems.

39. (B) Cultural competence.

This is the ability to demonstrate skills that facilitate communication and interaction between people with diverse ethnic values and religious beliefs.

40. (B) Suboptimal access to health care.

This factor is the most suitable answer to the high mortality rates among homeless patients. Factors that contribute to this include lack of access to health insurance, low socioeconomic status and instability.

41. (B) Educate her on the limitations of such treatment.

This intervention is most appropriate because the AG-ACNP is obligated to fulfill the role of an advocate and facilitator of learning. However, this must be done in an honest and non-confronting way that encourages collaboration and adherence.

42. (C) A 35-year-old Hispanic American.

Hispanic Americans are three times more likely to develop diabetes than non-Hispanic Americans.

43. (C) Insufficient instruction on treatment modalities.

This is a clinician barrier in patients' non-adherence. When patients are not properly educated on the significance of the treatment modalities, including the instructions they are to follow, they are likely to be complacent in their treatment.

44. (D) Bureaucracy and bottleneck.

Bureaucracy from administrative requirements can dissuade patients from seeking health care in the first place and keep them from sticking to the treatment plan.

45. (B) Sexual orientation.

Patients' sexual orientation does not prevent them from adhering to expert medical treatment. Economic status can prevent them from affording the cost of health care, which can, in turn, prevent them from seeking expert care; culture and ethnicity influence views on the causes and treatments of diseases; and family support can determine how cooperative a patient will be in sticking to treatment, especially when it is unpleasant.

46. (C) To assess the patient's sociocultural orientation.

This is not a good reason to obtain a detailed list of complementary therapies from a patient who is believed to be using supplemental herbs and remedies.

47. (D) Inform social services.

This response is inappropriate unless indicated. For example, a patient can insist on being discharged against medical advice for reasons that are not related to money or welfare. A patient may decide to be discharged for personal, religious and cultural reasons.

48. (C) Using the left hand to provide prescription notes.

In West African culture, using the left hand to provide materials is considered offensive.

49. (D) Refer her to a dietician.

This is the most appropriate intervention in ensuring that the patient loses weight permanently by making long-term dietary lifestyle changes. Options A and B are likely to work on a short-term basis but are largely unsuitable for long-term results. Option C is not effective for weight loss.

50. (C) Rotator cuff tears.

A classic sign of a rotator cuff tear is an exacerbation of shoulder pain when the affected joint is abducted or flexed at 60 to 120 degrees. However, the pain abates or is absent when the abduction/flexion is at an angle that is less than 60 degrees or more than 120 degrees.

51. (D) Impaired myocardial contractility.

Distributive shock occurs when there is massive arterial or venous dilation and a consequent drop in tissue perfusion. In this case, the circulating volume is normal. Causes include septic shock, neurogenic shock and poisoning from opioids, nitrates and B-blockers.

52. (B) Leukoplakia.

Leukoplakia is a white, flat-topped plaque that occurs due to chronic irritation of the oral mucosa. Risk factors include HIV, alcohol consumption, vitamin deficiencies and endocrine abnormalities.

53. (C) Phosphate enema.

A phosphate enema is the best choice for fecal impaction, not an oral laxative or a stool softener.

54. (B) L4.

The knee-jerk reflex is relayed by the L3 and L4 nerve root fibers.

55. (D) Impoverishment.

Organic causes of failure to thrive include acute and chronic disorders that affect intake, absorption, excretion and metabolism of food nutrients. Impoverishment is an example of an inorganic failure to thrive.

56. (A) Celiac disease.

This patient has malabsorption syndrome caused by celiac disease. Although the features of celiac disease are nonspecific and may overlap with features of other malabsorption syndromes, the presence of dermatitis herpetiformis is usually classic of celiac disease.

57. (B) Albendazole therapy.

This patient has Loeffler's syndrome secondary to Ascaris infection. Significant findings that support this diagnosis include a history of a recent trip to Asia, eosinophilia, chest symptoms and pulmonary infiltrates on a chest X-ray.

58. (B) Antitoxin to neutralize bound tetanospasmin.

This statement is incorrect because the anti-tetanus immunoglobulin neutralizes free-circulating toxins and not toxins that are already bound to the synaptic channels.

59. (D) A review of systems should include both nonspecific symptoms and system-specific symptoms.

Option A is incorrect because laboratory tests should not be requested without considering the possibility of the test showing different results. Option B is incorrect because there is a possibility of error of omission and missed diagnoses. Option C is incorrect because fever patterns are usually not required for diagnosing fever of unknown origin. Therefore, only option D is an appropriate treatment.

60. (A) Paget's disease of the breast.

Paget disease is breast carcinoma that looks like a unilateral eczematous lesion on the nipple and areola. It results from an extension to the epidermis of an underlying ductal adenocarcinoma of the breast. There should be a suspicion because the lesion is well delineated, unilateral and unresponsive to topical treatment.

61. (C) Colostomy.

This patient has metastatic spread to the colon. Definitive treatment is a palliative colostomy.

62. (A) Cholecystitis.

The most likely diagnosis is cholecystitis. The features in the history that support this diagnosis are that the patient is female, 45, and fertile.

63. (D) Digital rectal examination.

This patient has severe neutropenia, which is an emergency because he is both febrile and immunocompromised. To reduce the risk of gastrointestinal infections, digital rectal examination and/or the use of a rectal thermometer should be avoided.

64. (C) Oral nystatin suspension.

This patient has mucositis caused by radiation therapy. Treatment includes mouthwash with an analgesic before meals and avoidance of citrus juice and extremely hot and extremely cold foods. Feeding tubes may be used in extreme cases. Option C is incorrect because nystatin is used for oral candidiasis.

65. (D) Enema.

Patients with aplastic anemia are at an increased risk for bleeding (thrombocytopenia) and infections (neutropenia). Therefore enemas must be avoided as much as possible.

66. (D) Miosis.

Miosis is a feature of opioid intoxication, not withdrawal.

67. (D) The level of consciousness in delirium is more impaired than that in dementia.

This statement is false because the level of consciousness in delirium is typically impaired, while that of dementia is not usually impaired unless in severe cases.

68. (D) Hypothyroidism.

This is an adverse effect of long-term use of lithium, not a risk factor for lithium toxicity.

69. (B) A risk of suicidal ideas and attempts.

The FDA has warned that there is an increased risk of suicidal ideas and attempts in patients who are 24 years and below who are prescribed such medications. The guardians of this patient should be counseled to monitor her for increased agitation, depression and anxiousness within a week of commencement of the drug.

70. (B) Sertraline.

SSRIs, particularly sertraline, are the drug of choice for patients with ischemic heart disease because they have few cardiac conduction effects.

71. (C) Nasotracheal intubation.

Nasotracheal intubations can trigger coughing and gagging and further increase the ICP. Therefore, to intubate this patient, oral intubation should be used.

72. (C) Mannitol is given over 45 minutes.

This statement is false. Mannitol is an osmotic diuretic that is given to reduce ICP and maintain serum osmolality. It must be administered over 15 to 30 minutes as 2.5 to 2 ml/kg and repeated as 1.25 to 5 ml/kg every six to eight hours or as needed.

73. (D) Global hypertonia.

Global hypertonia is not a usual feature of meningitis. This patient is likely to demonstrate a positive Brudzinski's sign, which is described in Option A; a positive Kernig's sign, which is described in option B; and features of papilledema, which may indicate raised ICP.

74. (C) Palpate for the anterior superior iliac spine, which connects the two iliac crests across the L4 spinous process.

This statement is false because the landmark is the anterior iliac crest, which is an imaginary line that crosses the L4 spinous process.

75. (A) A preponderance of lymphocytes.

This is unlikely because the CSF analysis of bacterial meningitis is expected to reveal a great increase in the number of leucocytes (polymorphonuclear cells).

76. (D) Idiopathic intracranial hypertension.

The CSF analysis of this patient shows a raised intracranial pressure. However, the whole blood cell count, protein and glucose are all normal. In meningitis, the opening pressure is raised, glucose is depleted and protein is elevated. In cerebral hemorrhage, the opening pressure is increased and the glucose levels are normal, while the CSF protein is increased with a preponderance of red blood cells.

77. (C) Absence seizures.

Absence seizures/petit mal seizures manifest as a loss of consciousness that lasts for 10 to 30 seconds with associated eyelid fluttering. However, there is no loss of axial muscle tone, convulsions or postictal symptoms. The patient abruptly stops activity and resumes it with amnesia of the preceding events.

78. (D) General onset seizures.

General onset seizures are not a risk for relapse. Relapse is very likely in patients with any one of the following: a seizure disorder that started since childhood, a need for more than one anti-seizure drug, a history of seizures while taking an antiseizure drug, focal onset or myoclonic seizures, an underlying static encephalopathy, abnormal EEG result within the last year and the presence of structural brain lesions on imaging studies.

79. (C) Guillain-Barré syndrome.

This patient has the classic presentation of Guillain-Barré, which is a progressive flaccid weakness of the proximities that begins at the lower limbs and spreads to the arm, as well as paresthesia.

80. (B) Foot drop.

In this condition, the patient has a weakness of the affected foot and an inability to dorsiflex. Unilateral causes include peroneal nerve palsy and L5 radiculopathy.

81. (A) Ischemic stroke.

This patient has a hemiplegic gait that is commonly seen in stroke patients.

82. (A) Cerebral palsy.

This patient is displaying a diplegic gait that is caused by bilateral periventricular lesions.

83. (A) Muscular dystrophy.

This patient has a myopathic gait caused by weakness of the muscles of the hip girdle. He has bilateral weakness on both sides of the hip, causing him to waddle.

84. (B) Steven Johnson syndrome.

The features that confirm this diagnosis are a history of use of antiseizure drugs, widespread blisters that affect less than 20 percent of the body surface and involvement of mucocutaneous surfaces.

85. (C) Allergic contact dermatitis.

Features that support this diagnosis are the presence of erythema and vesicles that are arranged in a pattern. In this case, it is circumferential (around her wrist), meaning the allergic reaction was triggered by jewelry.

86. (C) Pityriasis rubra pilaris.

This is a chronic skin disorder that causes hyperkeratosis of the trunk and extremities, particularly the palms and soles. Most particularly, red follicular papules coalesce into scaling plaques with islands of normal skin between them.

87. (B) eGFR 60 to 89.

Stage-2 kidney disease is characterized by an estimated glomerular filtration rate of 60 to 89.

88. (C) Nonionic contrast agents.

Nonionic contrast agents with lower osmolality (500 to 850 mOsm/kg) have a lower risk of causing nephrotoxicity compared to ionic agents with a high osmolality of 1,400 to 1,800 mOsm/kg.

89. (B) Serum creatinine.

In contrast nephropathy, there is a progressive increase in serum creatinine 24 to 48 hours after a contrast study.

90. (B) Analgesic nephropathy.

This patient has the classic features of analgesic nephropathy: hematuria, flank pain, dyspepsia, hypertension, anemia, joint pain, headaches and impaired ability to concentrate urine.

91. (B) Prostatic cancer.

This patient has bladder outlet obstruction that is secondary to prostate cancer. The DRE findings of prostate cancer are stony, hard nodules that extend to the seminal vesicles, fixing of the prostate to the lateral wall and extension of the gland through the capsule.

92. (A) Paralytic ileus.

This is a cause of hypokalemia. Protracted vomiting can lead to loss of H ions, metabolic alkalosis and subsequent renal losses of potassium.

93. (B) IV calcium gluconate.

Although hemodialysis is indicated in this patient, IV calcium gluconate should be promptly administered to stabilize the cardiac cells and reduce the risk of arrhythmia.

94. (D) Anorectal fissure.

An anorectal fissure is a cause of lower GI bleeding.

95. (D) Spoon-shaped nails.

This is not a typical feature of chronic liver disease. Spoon-shaped nails are seen in iron-deficiency anemia and hemosiderosis.

96. (A) Gastric carcinoma.

Features of early gastric cancer are nonspecific. However, as the disease progresses, specific abnormalities include an epigastric mass; umbilical, left supraclavicular, left axillary lymph nodes; hepatomegaly and ovarian or rectal masses.

97. (A) Bloating.

The left colon is narrower than the right colon. Therefore, symptoms of the left colon are obstructive symptoms, like bloating, constipation, diarrhea, abdominal cramps, abdominal distension, nausea and vomiting. Symptoms of right-sided colon cancer are features of chronic anemia and hematemesis.

98. (A) Cirrhosis.

This patient has features of alcoholic liver disease. Although the clinical features of cirrhosis are the same as the other diseases described, on examination of the liver, the liver is typically shrunken in cirrhosis.

99. (B) Opioids are useful for advanced cases of alcoholic liver disease.

This statement is false because excess sedation with opioids can trigger portal encephalopathy and coma. As such, opioids are generally avoided in advanced cases.

100. (D) Use of intravenous potassium.

Massive blood transfusion is the replacement of more than 50 percent of the total body blood volume in four hours or the replacement of more than one blood volume in 24 hours. The complications of massive blood transfusion include hyperkalemia. Therefore, the use of intravenous potassium is contraindicated.

101. (C) Post-transfusion purpura.

This is a late-onset reaction that usually occurs about four to 14 days after a blood transfusion. The platelet count begins to fall steadily, causing moderate to severe thrombocytopenia.

102. (C) Examples include urticaria.

Type 1 hypersensitivity reaction is also called an immediate hypersensitivity reaction. It is IgE-mediated. Examples include most atopic and allergic reactions, like allergic rhinitis, asthma, urticaria, angioedema and allergic reactions to venomous stings.

103. (B) Type II.

Type II hypersensitivity reactions are also called antibody-dependent cytotoxic hypersensitivity reactions. They occur when an antibody binds to an antigen to form an antibody-antigen complex that activates antibody-dependent cell-mediated inflammation.

104. (D) IV atenolol.

This patient has anaphylaxis. Management includes oxygen and ventilator support, vasoconstrictors like epinephrine, nebulized bronchodilators and IV hydrocortisone. IV atenolol is a beta-blocker whose use is not only irrelevant but also harmful in this patient, who already has bronchoconstriction.

105. (D) Peripheral neuropathy.

This is not an example of a drug hypersensitivity reaction. Examples of drug hypersensitivity reactions include serum sickness, drug-induced hemolytic anemia; drug rashes with eosinophilia and systemic symptoms; drug-induced pulmonary disease, including interstitial lung disease; tubo-interstitial nephritis; SLE like syndromes and others.

106. (C) Addison's disease

This patient has the classic features of an adrenal crisis in Addison's disease. The features are hyperpigmentation of the mucous membranes and pressure areas of the body, profound weakness and hypokalemia.

107. (D) ACTH stimulation test.

ACTH stimulation test is used to diagnose Addison's disease, not Cushing.

108. (B) Excess secretion of ACTH from a non-pituitary tumor.

The other options are examples of Cushing syndrome. Cushing's disease is a primary disorder caused by excessive production of pituitary ACTH. Cushing syndrome is caused by an endogenous/exogenous secretion of cortisol.

109. (B) Insulin therapy when potassium is 3 mmol/L.

Insulin therapy must be withheld until the serum potassium is greater than or equal to 3.3 mmol/L. Insulin can cause an uptake of K into the cells, further depleting serum potassium levels.

110. (C) Hyperglycemia.

Hyperglycemia is not a feature of alcoholic ketoacidosis. Alcohol depletes the glucose in the liver, stimulates the action of gluconeogenic hormones, decreases insulin secretion and increases lipolysis. This causes an elevated anion gap metabolic acidosis. Plasma glucose levels are either low or normal. They are slightly high in a few cases.

111. (A) There is an insufficient secretion of vasopressin.

Nephrogenic diabetes insipidus is characterized by an inability to concentrate urine, even in the presence of vasopressin.

112. (C) Elevated alveolar hydrostatic pressure.

This patient has acute respiratory failure caused by left ventricular failure. In this case, there is an increase in the hydrostatic pressure of the alveoli and consequent flooding of the lungs.

113. (C) Mechanical ventilation.

This patient most likely has acute respiratory failure caused by pneumonia. Although antipyretics are used for controlling the fever, and an emergency chest X-ray diagnoses the cause of the respiratory failure, it is important that this patient first receive assisted ventilatory support to reduce the risk of cardiopulmonary failure and death.

114. (D) Using nasal prongs for improved oxygen delivery.

This treatment is inappropriate because nasal prongs are not used for mechanical ventilation. Materials used for mechanical ventilation are endotracheal tubes, oropharyngeal and nasopharyngeal airway tubes.

115. (C) Pneumothorax.

This patient has pneumothorax. The clinical features are decreased breath sounds, tactile fremitus on the affected area and hyperresonant sounds on percussion. If the pneumothorax is large enough, there will be a shifting of the trachea to the contralateral side.

116. (A) Subcutaneous emphysema.

This patient most likely has a pneumomediastinum caused by a rupture of the alveoli. Chest X-ray findings include air in the mediastinum, subcutaneous emphysema, double bronchial sign and continuous diaphragm sign.

117. (B) Emergency thoracocentesis.

This patient has a tension pneumothorax and is at risk of shock. An emergency thoracocentesis should be performed even without confirming the diagnosis with a chest X-ray.

118. (B) Secure an airway with an endotracheal tube.

This patient has angioedema and is at risk of cardiopulmonary failure from airway obstruction. The most important step is to secure an airway for assisted ventilation before commencing other supportive management and treating the underlying cause.

119. (C) Chest X-ray.

This patient most likely has a spontaneous pneumothorax from a bulla. Men with a tall, thin habitus are at risk of having this.

120. (D) Obstructive sleep apnea.

This patient most likely has obstructive sleep apnea that affected his concentration at work and led to the fracture. The clinical features of obstructive sleep apnea include hypersomnolence, fatigue, morning headaches, dry mouth and impaired concentration. The patient may not notice initial symptoms like snoring, gasping and choking during sleep.

121. (C) Sleep studies.

This patient has obstructive sleep apnea. Diagnostic tests include sleep studies that are used for symptom criteria. Confirmatory diagnosis is polysomnography.

122. (C) Bronchogenic CA.

This patient most likely has a bronchogenic carcinoma. The absence of a chronic cough and night sweats rules out pulmonary tuberculosis, while the absence of a productive cough rules out COPD.

123. (D) Mucus plugs.

Mucus plugs are not a feature of emphysema. This is because a productive cough is not a usual feature of emphysema. A productive cough is typically seen in chronic bronchitis.

124. (B) Cor pulmonale.

This patient has right ventricular failure caused by a disorder of the lungs and the vasculature. In this case, there is a dilatation of the capillary beds in the alveoli caused by bullous changes.

125. (C) It is indicated for patients with less than 50% occlusion.

This is false. Percutaneous coronary intervention (PCI) is contraindicated in patients with less than 50 percent occlusion. Other contraindications include total occlusion of the coronary artery, hypercoagulable states, diffused diseased vessels without focal stenosis and the presence of a singular diseased vessel that provides sole perfusion to the myocardium.

126. (A) A 58-year-old man with hypercholesterolemia and dyspnea on exertion.

Stress testing is used to diagnose CAD in patients with identified risks. It is also used to monitor patients with CAD. The other patients are unfit for a stress test.

127. (C) Primary Reynaud's syndrome.

This patient meets the criteria for primary Reynaud's syndrome. These criteria include symmetric attacks on both hands, no tissue necrosis or gangrene and age of onset that is less than 40 years.

128. (C) Congestive heart failure.

Congestive heart failure is a cause of cardiogenic shock, not distributive shock. In distributive shock, arterial or venous vasodilation causes tissue hypoperfusion.

129. (D) Increased coronary artery perfusion.

In atrial fibrillation, the most appropriate immediate intervention is to increase perfusion of the cardiomyocytes and decrease cardiac demand by placing the patient on bed rest. Thrombolytic therapy is not typically indicated for atrial fibrillation, nor is decreasing cardiac output and anxiolytic therapy.

130. (A) Tall tented T waves.

The ECG findings in hyperkalemia include tall tented T waves, which is the earliest sign; widened and flattened P wave; broad PR segment; flattened P wave and widened QRS complex.

131. (C) Hypokalemia.

The ECG findings in hypokalemia include a widened P wave with prolonged PR interval, flattening and depression of the T waves, ST depression, prominent U waves and long QU interval.

132. (D) Wolff-Parkinson-White syndrome.

The classic findings of this syndrome in sinus rhythm include a shortened PR interval that is less than 120 m, the presence of a delta wave, prolongation of the QRS complex that is more than 110 ms and discordant changes in the ST segment and T wave.

133. (D) The T wave lasts for approximately 270 ms.

This statement is false because the T wave, which represents ventricular diastole, lasts for about 430 ms. Ventricular diastole is divided into two phases. In phase 1, the ventricular muscles relax, and pressure within the ventricle falls. The semilunar valves are then closed to prevent the backflow of blood into the heart. In phase 2, the ventricles relax and pressure drops until it becomes lower than the pressure in the atria. This pushes the tricuspid and mitral valves open.

134. (C) The anterior wall.

In ECG, the anterior wall of the heart is represented by the anterior leads, which is V1 to V6, and the inferior wall is represented by leads II, III and aVF. The posterior wall is represented by the right anterior leads.

135. (A) Pharmacological intervention is with beta-blockers, calcium channel blockers and diuretics.

Diuretics, nitrates and ACE inhibitors are contraindicated for patients with hypertrophic cardiomyopathy. Since the underlying pathology is in the diastolic function, and systolic function is preserved, reducing the arterial resistance has no therapeutic benefit.

136. (C) Spironolactone is an ACE inhibitor and a potassium-sparing diuretic.

Spironolactone is an aldosterone antagonist. Examples of ACE inhibitors are lisinopril and enalapril.

137. (B) It is a potassium-sparing diuretic.

Furosemide is a loop diuretic that is used to reduce volume overload and subsequent preload on the heart. It is a potassium-wasting drug. Hypokalemia, hyponatremia and hypophosphatemia are side effects of its use.

138. (B) A 55-year-old woman with chronic atrial arrhythmia.

Digoxin is not useful in patients with diastolic heart failure or who are in acute heart failure. However, digoxin may be beneficial for patients with chronic arrhythmia and systolic heart failure.

139. (C) Pedal edema is a side effect of amlodipine.

Amlodipine is a calcium channel blocker used to decrease high blood pressure and reduce the risk of angina. However, it cannot be used to treat already-occurring angina. Side effects include pedal edema, headaches, flushes, constipation, palpitations and others.

140. (D) Digoxin.

Digoxin is inappropriate and even harmful in patients with hypertrophic cardiomyopathy because this is a disease of diastolic dysfunction.

141. (A) Digoxin toxicity.

Visual disturbance is a sign of digoxin toxicity. Severe signs are ventricular tachycardia and fibrillation.

142. (C) Intravenous furosemide.

This patient has pulmonary edema caused by left ventricular heart failure. Treatment includes administration of oxygen, administration of an IV diuretic to provide prompt relief from pulmonary congestion, pain relief, control of blood pressure and commencement of heart failure management.

143. (D) Administration of oxygen.

This patient's respiratory function is suboptimal, placing him at risk for cardiopulmonary failure. The first response should be to administer oxygen. Thereafter, IV antipyretics can be given, and a chest X-ray can be done to confirm pleural effusion.

144. (D) Give supplemental oxygen.

This patient has angina pectoris caused by myocardial infarction (MI). During MI, there is decreased oxygen perfusion to the myocardium, triggering ischemic pain and vasospasm. Oxygen should be administered before administering nitroglycerin and morphine. An ECG is then done to diagnose MI.

145. (B) Stop digoxin.

Visual disturbance is a feature of digoxin toxicity. Other features include anorexia, nausea, vomiting and palpitations. Severe toxicity can lead to ventricular tachycardia and fibrillation. If a patient shows signs of toxicity, digoxin must be stopped immediately, and electrolytes must be monitored and corrected for any imbalance.

146. (C) Echocardiography.

This man has a valvular disease, most likely stenosis of the aortic valve, which is commonly seen in the elderly. Echocardiography is diagnostic of the condition.

147. (D) Imagination.

The mini-mental state exam is used to assess a patient's cognition. Components of this exam include orientation, registration, attention, recall, language and copying. Imagination is not a component of the exam.

148. (B) Take this paper, fold it in two and give it to me.

Option B assesses the patient's language skills. Option A assesses orientation. Option C assesses copying, and Option D assesses attention.

149. (D) There are six Korotkoff sounds.

This statement is incorrect because there are five Korotkoff sounds. They are phase I, which is a thud; phase II, which is a blowing noise; phase III, which is a softer thud than in phase I; phase IV, which is a disappearing blowing noise and phase V, which is silent.

150. (D) Percussion for cardiac size.

This answer is incorrect because cardiac percussion is not part of the cardiovascular exam. To assess the size of the heart, the location of the apex beat is done via palpation.

Test 3: Questions

1. Patient M is a 65-year-old patient being managed for left ventricular heart failure. Which of the following findings is least likely to be seen on a chest X-ray?

    A. Washed cardiac silhouette
    B. Pleural effusion
    C. Kerley B lines
    D. Flattened hemi-diaphragms

2. Patient F is a known hypertensive who presents to the ER with complaints of dyspnea, chest pain, restlessness and cyanosis. An urgent chest X-ray shows blunting of the left costophrenic angle. Which of the following best explains the reason for the condition?

    A. Increased capillary hydrostatic pressure
    B. Decreased plasma oncotic pressure
    C. Increased capillary permeability
    D. Massive hemothorax

3. Which of the following drugs is inappropriate for a patient with diastolic heart failure?

    A. ACE inhibitor
    B. ARBs
    C. Beta-blockers
    D. Diuretics

4. Patient V just had prosthetic valve surgery for valvular stenosis. Which of the following statements is false?

    A. The patient should inform health personnel of his heart valve before dental procedures are performed.
    B. Regular monitoring of his clotting profile is required.
    C. Pulmonary hypertension is a complication of his condition.
    D. Prompt commencement of chest physiotherapy is called for.

5. Patient M is a 68-year-old male who complains of palpitations. ECG shows an irregular sinus rhythm. Heart rate is 150 bpm. BP is 130/80 mmHg. There are no signs of heart failure or myocardial ischemia. Which of the following drugs is suitable?

A. Digoxin
B. Enalapril
C. Atenolol
D. Losartan

6. A 30-year-old cyclist is admitted to the ER with a penetrating injury to the chest. On examination, there is dyspnea; his trachea is central; his external jugular veins are distended, and there are absent breath sounds and hyperresonant notes on the left hemithorax. Which of the following diagnoses is appropriate?

A. Cardiac tamponade
B. Flail chest
C. Tension pneumothorax
D. Massive hemothorax

7. A patient presents to the ER with complaints of recurrent breathlessness, chest pain and increased anxiety. On examination, there are visible and distended neck veins, abdominal pain in the upper right quadrant and pedal edema. A history of mitral valve replacement is also obtained. A cardiac examination reveals a holosystolic murmur. Which is the most appropriate diagnosis?

A. Mitral stenosis
B. Mitral regurgitation
C. Tricuspid regurgitation
D. Aortic stenosis

8. A 45-year-old woman is rushed to the ER with complaints of difficulty in breathing, chest pain and restlessness. On examination, BP is 100/80 mmHg, PR is 120 bpm and BMI is 26 kg/m2. Which of the following diagnoses is appropriate?

A. Pulmonary edema
B. Pulmonary embolism
C. Pleural effusion
D. Hemothorax

9. A 58-year-old male presents to the ER with chest pain, diaphoresis and syncope. On examination, PR is 120 bpm and BP is 140/100 mmHg. ECG shows an ST elevation. Which of the following interventions is definitive?

    A. Beta-blockers
    B. Thrombolytics
    C. Percutaneous angiography
    D. Aspirin

10. Patient M is a 55-year-old female being worked up for contrast angiography of the coronary arteries. Which of the following is necessary for renal protection?

    A. IV Lasix
    B. 0.9% saline
    C. Ringer's lactate
    D. 5% dextrose saline

11. Patient M is being worked up for contrast angiography of her coronary arteries. Which of the following principles is incorrect?

    A. Hydrate with normal saline 24 hours before the procedure.
    B. Diabetes mellitus is a risk factor for contrast nephropathy.
    C. Ionic contrast agents are hypo osmolar to the blood.
    D. Patients with asthma are at risk of allergic-type contrast reactions.

12. What is the ideal antihypertensive for an Afro Caribbean who has a blood pressure of 150/100 mmHg and no other complications?

    A. Losartan
    B. Enalapril
    C. Amlodipine
    D. Methyldopa

13. A 45-year-old patient presents to the ER with complaints of occasional episodes of difficulty breathing and diaphoresis. She says that the severity of the chest pain has been increasing in intensity with each episode. Which of the following diagnoses is most appropriate?

    A. Stable angina
    B. Unstable angina
    C. Myocardial infarction
    D. Aortic stenosis

14. Patient O is a 55-year-old female on amlodipine and enalapril. She complains of falls and dizziness. Which of the following investigations is most appropriate?

   A. Head CT scan
   B. Echocardiogram
   C. ECG
   D. 24-hour BP monitoring

15. A 24-year-old basketball varsity athlete suddenly slumps during a basketball game. Which of the following is the most likely cause?

   A. Myocardial infarction
   B. Hypertrophic cardiomyopathy
   C. Valvular heart disorder
   D. Cardiac tamponade

16. Patient Y is a 56-year-old white male who is a recently diagnosed diabetic hypertensive. Which of the following antihypertensives is suitable?

   A. Amlodipine
   B. Lisinopril
   C. Nifedipine
   D. Thiazide

17. Patient M is a 75-year-old male with hypertension. He has just been diagnosed with prostate cancer. An ultrasound of the urinary system and prostate shows bilaterally shrunken kidneys and an enlarged prostate. Which of the following best explains the pathology in the kidneys?

   A. Metastatic infiltration to the kidneys
   B. Hypertensive kidney disease
   C. Chronic glomerulonephritis
   D. Renal agenesis

18. Patient M presents to the ER with altered sensorium, agitation and motor and sensory deficit on the left lower and upper limbs. The blood pressure on presentation is 220/120 mmHg. Which of the following anti-hypertensives is appropriate in controlling the blood pressure?

A. Labetalol
B. Nifedipine
C. Sublingual nitroglycerin
D. Amlodipine

19. Patient G is a 55-year-old hypertensive on spironolactone, losartan and lisinopril. He complains of increased breast tissue. Which of the following interventions is appropriate?

A. Reduce losartan dosage
B. Stop spironolactone
C. Stop losartan
D. Encourage the patient to continue his medication

20. Patient G is a 55-year-old hypertensive who presents to the ER with complaints of palpitations, numbness and nausea. Her electrolyte results are as follows: Na 135 mEq/L, K 5.5 mEq/L, Urea 10 mmol/L, creatinine 70 umol/L. She is currently on spironolactone, losartan and captopril. Which of the following interventions is appropriate?

A. Stop losartan.
B. Stop spironolactone.
C. Stop captopril.
D. Commence hemodialysis.

21. Which of the following positions is appropriate for securing the airway in a patient with a suspected cervical injury?

A. Supine position
B. Sniffling position
C. Probe position
D. High Fowler's

22. A 46-year-old male is rushed to the ER with shortness of breath, coughing and hemoptysis. On examination, there is tachycardia, tachypnea and stridor. SP02 in atmospheric oxygen is 86%, and the patient is noted to be markedly wasted. Which of the following interventions is appropriate?

    A. Emergency chest X-ray
    B. Emergency bronchoscopy
    C. Emergency tracheostomy
    D. Emergency thoracostomy

23. You are managing a patient with a chronic cough that is productive of thick and purulent sputum. The patient also has dyspnea, wheezing and finger clubbing. Chest X-ray findings include linear perihilar densities and tram lines. What is the most appropriate diagnosis?

    A. Chronic bronchitis
    B. Emphysema
    C. Bronchiectasis
    D. Interstitial lung disease

24. Which of the following best defines an exacerbation of bronchiectasis?

    A. Deterioration of clinical symptoms lasting for at least 48 hours
    B. Deterioration of clinical symptoms lasting for at least 24 hours
    C. Deterioration of clinical symptoms lasting for at least 36 hours
    D. Deterioration of clinical symptoms lasting for at least 72 hours

25. Which of the following statements best describes the etiology of primary pulmonary hypertension?

    A. Right ventricular failure caused by a disorder of the lung vasculature
    B. Right-to-left shunting of blood
    C. Increased alveolar pressure caused by alveolar dead space
    D. Pulmonary vascular hypertrophy

26. Which of the following is not useful in the management of the patient with cor pulmonale secondary to COPD?

    A. Pulmonary vasodilators
    B. Diuretics
    C. Oxygen therapy
    D. IV antibiotics

27. A 35-year-old female presents to the ER with shortness of breath, fatigue and chest pain. On general examination, the patient looks toxic, temperature is 38°C. RR is 40 cpm. PR is 100 bpm. BP is 110/80 mmHg. On chest examination, there is reduced chest expansion, and there are decreased resonant sounds and bronchial breath sounds on the right hemithorax. Which of the following statements is false?

    A. A chest X-ray is likely to show lobar infiltrates on the right hemithorax.
    B. A chest X-ray is likely to show subpleural reticular opacities.
    C. Broad-spectrum antibiotics may be useful.
    D. The patient may be immunosuppressed.

28. Which of the following organisms is not implicated in atypical pneumonia?

    A. Cryptococcus spp
    B. Mycoplasma spp
    C. Moraxella catarrhalis
    D. Legionnaires' disease

29. A 55-year-old patient has been stable on a mechanical ventilator for the past three days. During the rounds, you notice that the patient is tachycardic, tachypneic and febrile. During suctioning, you observe that the secretions are purulent and offensive. Which of the following diagnoses is most accurate?

    A. Pneumothorax
    B. Ventilator-associated pneumonia
    C. Hospital-acquired pneumonia
    D. Atypical pneumonia

30. You have just intubated a patient for mechanical ventilation. Which of the following measures is not useful in reducing the risk for ventilator-associated pneumonia?

    A. Positioning the patient in the recumbent position
    B. Ventilation with a CPAP or BiPAP
    C. Continuous aspiration of subglottic secretions
    D. Prompt weaning off the ventilator as soon as indicated

31. A patient with HIV stage 3 presents to the ER with complaints of a dry, non-productive cough that has lasted for weeks and associated shortness of breath. Chest X-ray findings show diffuse bilateral perihilar infiltrates. Which of the following pharmacological interventions is most appropriate?

A. Rifampicin and ethambutol
B. Vancomycin
C. Amphotericin B
D. Trimethoprim/sulfamethoxazole

32. M is a homeless 28-year-old male who presents to the ER with chronic productive cough, hemoptysis and fever. On examination, he is markedly wasted with cervical lymphadenopathy. Which of the following tests is inappropriate for diagnosis?

A. Chest X-ray
B. Acid-fast stain
C. Nucleic acid-based test
D. Blood culture

33. A patient on anti-Koch's therapy complains of seeing objects in washed-out/gray color. Which of the following drugs is implicated?

A. Rifampicin
B. Pyrazinamide
C. Ethambutol
D. Isoniazid

34. A 56-year-old male presents to the ER with worsening shortness of breath, dyspnea and cough that is productive of a tablespoonful of sputum. FEV1/FVC ratio before salbutamol is 64%. FEV1/FVC ratio 20 minutes after salbutamol is 65%. Which of the following is the most appropriate diagnosis?

A. Asthma
B. Chronic bronchitis
C. Lung fibrosis
D. Bronchiectasis

35. A known asthmatic presents to the ER with exacerbated symptoms of asthma. After administration of oxygen, nebulized salbutamol and hydrocortisone, symptoms do not improve. The nebulized bronchodilator is re-administered with IV magnesium sulfate. Arterial blood gas shows paO2 45 mmHg. Which of the following interventions is most appropriate?

    A. Noninvasive positive pressure ventilation
    B. Mechanical ventilation
    C. IV diazepam
    D. IV Augmentin

36. A 62-year-old male presents to the ER with complaints of chest pain and breathlessness. A history of progressive weight loss and occupation as a home construction worker is obtained. An emergency chest X-ray shows bilateral fibrosis and left-sided pleural effusion. Which of the following investigations is most appropriate?

    A. Pleural fluid cytology
    B. Pleural biopsy
    C. MRI
    D. CT pulmonary angiography

37. A homeless woman is admitted to the ER with altered sensorium, fever, fast breathing and chronic cough productive of foul-smelling sputum. On examination, PR is 100 bpm, RR is 35 cpm, temperature is 39°C and there are hyporesonant notes on the left hemithorax. She is noted to have dental caries. An emergency chest X-ray shows cavitary lesions in the lungs. Which of the following diagnoses is most appropriate?

    A. Pulmonary tuberculosis
    B. Empyema
    C. Chronic bronchitis
    D. Bronchiectasis

38. A group of young adults is admitted to the ER with altered consciousness, diaphoresis and seizures. Significant findings on examination include tachycardia and pyrexia. A history of MDMA use is obtained. Which of the following electrolyte imbalances is most likely?

    A. Hyponatremia
    B. Hypernatremia
    C. Hypokalemia
    D. Hyperkalemia

39. Patient M is a 55-year-old female who is currently being managed for primary hypothyroidism. Which of the following statements is false?

   A. Serum T3 is very sensitive for screening.
   B. TSH is usually elevated.
   C. Serum-free T4 and T3 are low.
   D. Microcytic hypochromic anemia is a usual finding.

40. Which of the following pharmacological interventions is suitable for a patient with thyroid storm?

   A. Radioactive iodine
   B. Methimazole
   C. Propylthiouracil
   D. Iodine

41. A patient with thyroid storm has just been given IV propranolol. Which of the following symptoms is unlikely to respond to propranolol?

   A. Tachycardia
   B. Heart intolerance
   C. Exophthalmos
   D. Proximal neuropathy

42. Concerning the principles of pharmacological interventions for hyperthyroidism, which of the following statements is false?

   A. Iodine inhibits the release of T3 and T4.
   B. Methimazole blocks the action of thyroid peroxidase.
   C. Agranulocytosis is an adverse effect of propylthiouracil.
   D. Methimazole is readily converted to carbimazole.

43. Which of the following is not an indication for thyroidectomy?

   A. Large goiter with compression syndrome
   B. Toxic adenoma
   C. Multinodular goiter
   D. Thyrotoxicosis

44. A 50-year-old woman presents to the ER with headache, dizziness, tinnitus and visual disturbances. She also gives a history of pruritus on the hands and toes after a hot shower. Significant findings on examination include splenomegaly. Hematologic labs reveal RBC 87, Hgb 31.9, Plt 796. What is the most appropriate diagnosis?

    A. CML
    B. Polycythemia rubra
    C. Myelofibrosis
    D. Non-Hodgkin's lymphoma

45. A 65-year-old male presents to the ER with dizziness, shortness of breath, body weakness and fever. Significant findings on examination reveal purpuric rashes on his trunk and lower limbs, lymphadenopathy and hepatosplenomegaly. Which of the following is most likely to be seen on peripheral blood film?

    A. Reticulocytes
    B. Blast cells
    C. Inclusion bodies
    D. Megakaryocytes

46. Which of the following is not a significant feature of Hodgkin's lymphoma?

    A. Painless adenopathy
    B. Splenomegaly
    C. Hepatomegaly
    D. Unintentional weight loss

47. Which of the following is a confirmatory investigation for multiple myeloma?

    A. Complete blood count
    B. Protein electrophoresis
    C. Serum lactate dehydrogenase assay
    D. Bone X-ray

48. Which of the following is not a cause of secondary hemochromatosis?

    A. Sickle cell anemia
    B. Myelodysplasia
    C. G6PD deficiency
    D. Ferroportin disease

49. Which of the following is not an indication of cryoprecipitate transfusion?

    A. Massive transfusion
    B. Von Willebrand disease
    C. Acute DIC bleeding
    D. HELLP syndrome

50. A 55-year-old patient with decompensated liver disease is being managed for upper GI bleeding. After commencing resuscitation, endoscopic banding and IV octreotide are given. However, hematochezia persists. Which of the following interventions is appropriate?

    A. TIPS procedure
    B. Mechanical compression with Sengstaken-Blakemore tube
    C. Splenectomy
    D. Liver transplantation

51. A 66-year-old patient is being managed for decompensated liver failure secondary to alcoholic liver disease. Which of the following measures will not be useful in reducing the risk of hepatic encephalopathy?

    A. Bowel cleansing with oral lactulose
    B. Use of oral neomycin
    C. Providing a protein-free diet
    D. Avoiding sedatives and opioids

52. A patient with jaundice is being managed for acute liver hepatitis. Which of the following statements is correct?

    A. This is a form of unconjugated hyperbilirubinemia.
    B. Bilirubin is excreted in the urine
    C. Bilirubin is about 23 to 51 umol/L.
    D. Pruritus is an unusual feature.

53. What is the pathophysiology of GERD?

    A. Relaxation of the lower esophageal sphincter
    B. Protrusion of the stomach through a diaphragmatic hiatus
    C. A mucosal growth in the lumen of the esophagus
    D. Narrowing of the esophageal lumen

54. A 25-year-old female presents to the ER with altered consciousness, fever, diarrhea and vomiting. Significant findings on examination include BP 100/60 mmHg, PR 100 bpm, temp 38°C. Her stools are also found to be bloody. Which of the following interventions is inappropriate?

    A. Ringer's lactate
    B. Ciprofloxacin
    C. Loperamide
    D. Promethazine

55. A 22-year-old female presents to the ER with abdominal pain on defecation. There is a history of recurrent constipation alternating with diarrhea. Which of the following diagnoses is most likely?

    A. Malabsorption syndrome
    B. IBS
    C. Ulcerative colitis
    D. Colorectal cancer

56. A 25-year-old female is admitted to the ER with altered sensorium and seizures. A history of chronic use of water pills and laxatives for weight loss is collected. Biochemical tests reveal potassium 4.5 mmol/L, sodium 115 mmol/L, bicarbonate 22 mmol/L. Which of the following interventions is most appropriate?

    A. Administration of dextrose saline
    B. Administration of Ringer's lactate
    C. Use of vasopressin antagonist
    D. Use of hypertonic 3% saline

57. Which of the following is not a cause of hypovolemic hypernatremia?

    A. Diabetes mellitus
    B. Diuretics
    C. Chronic kidney disease
    D. Central diabetes insipidus

58. A patient has just been placed on urethral catheterization for chronic urinary retention caused by benign prostatic hyperplasia. Which of the following interventions is not useful in reducing the risk of catheter-associated urinary tract infections?

    A. Maintaining a closed drainage system
    B. Starting prostatectomy as soon as possible
    C. Prophylactic antibiotics
    D. Aseptic catheter insertion

59. A 19-year-old female presents to the ER with lower abdominal pain, fatigue and fever. Significant findings on examination include cervical motion tenderness. Which of the following organisms is not a cause?

    A. Chlamydia
    B. Gonorrhea
    C. Candida
    D. Trichomoniasis

60. A 56-year-old textile worker presents to the ER with gross painless hematuria, dizziness and fatigue. Significant findings include a palpable suprapubic mass. Which of the following diagnoses is most likely?

    A. Schistosomiasis
    B. Bladder cancer
    C. Prostate cancer
    D. Cystitis

61. A 25-year-old man presents to the ER with acute urinary retention. On examination, significant findings include a palpable suprapubic mass and suprapubic tenderness. Attempts at urethral catheterization are unsuccessful, so an emergency cysto catheterization is performed. Which of the following investigations confirms the diagnosis?

    A. Prostate ultrasound
    B. Abdominopelvic ultrasound
    C. Intravenous urography
    D. Retrograde urethrography

62. A 35-year-old male presents to the ER with severe scrotal pain, scrotal swelling, nausea and vomiting. Scrotal examination reveals edema of the left scrotum with testicular tenderness and absent cremasteric reflex in the left testis. The left testis is also tender and elevated. Which of the following diagnoses is appropriate?

A. Testicular cancer
B. Strangulated hernia
C. Testicular torsion
D. Varicocele

63. A 65-year-old woman presents to the ER with abdominal pain and persistent vomiting. On examination, there is an irreducible inguinal mass, rebound tenderness and guarding. Which of the following interventions is definitive?

A. Herniorrhaphy
B. Appendectomy
C. Exploratory laparotomy
D. Herniotomy

64. A 65-year-old female is admitted with intense itching and fever. Significant findings on examination include fluid-filled vesicles that are greater than 10 mm in diameter on the trunk and extensor surfaces of the upper and lower limbs. The Nikolsky sign is negative. Which of the following diagnoses is most appropriate?

A. Dermatitis herpetiformis
B. Bullous pemphigoid
C. Pemphigus vulgaris
D. Pemphigoid foliaceous

65. A 52-year-old female is admitted with a tenderness of the left leg and fever. Significant findings on examination include the warmth of the surrounding skin, erythema and peau d' orange of the affected skin. Which of the following diagnoses is most likely?

A. Deep vein thrombosis
B. Compartment syndrome
C. Cellulitis
D. Stasis dermatitis

66. A 25-year-old male presents with a history of red patches on his knees, elbows and scalp. He says that these lesions are episodic and non-pruritic. Significant findings on examination are well-demarcated lesions with silvery scales. There is minimal to no itching. Which of the following is most likely to be the cause?

- A. Hypersensitivity reaction
- B. Exposure to caustic substances
- C. Malassezia furfur
- D. Autoimmune reaction

67. A patient is admitted with nocturnal back pain, fatigue and weight loss. Significant findings on examination include pallor and diminished chest expansion. Which of the following diagnoses is most appropriate?

- A. Psoriatic arthritis
- B. Ankylosing spondylitis
- C. Rheumatoid arthritis
- D. Pott's disease

68. A 55-year-old male has dactylitis of the DIP joints of the left fingers and right elbow joint. Significant findings include erythematous papules with silvery scales on the scalp and gluteal folds. Which of the following diagnoses is most likely?

- A. SLE
- B. Psoriatic arthritis
- C. Metastatic melanoma
- D. Rheumatoid arthritis

69. A patient who is being managed for rheumatoid arthritis will benefit from all these DMARDs except:

- A. Methotrexate
- B. Celecoxib
- C. Leflunomide
- D. Hydroxychloroquine

70. A multi-trauma patient who is being managed in the ER begins to produce reddish-brown urine. Which of the following interventions is necessary?

    A. Order a serum creatinine kinase assay.
    B. Order a urine MCS.
    C. Commence platelet therapy.
    D. Perform an emergency fasciotomy.

71. A 56-year-old female presents to the ER with fatigue, a throbbing headache in the temporal region, scalp pain and double vision. Significant findings on examination include prominent temporal arteries, with erythema on the overlying skin. Hematologic investigations reveal an elevated ESR and C-reactive protein. Which of the following diagnoses is most likely?

    A. Bechet's disease
    B. Giant cell arteritis
    C. Polyarteritis nodosa
    D. Cutaneous vasculitis

72. A patient complains of headaches in the left temporal region that occur during the waking hours of the morning. Headaches are typically associated with restlessness, lacrimation and nasal congestion. The headaches are reported to subside about 40 minutes after onset. Which of the following diagnoses is most accurate?

    A. Tension-type headache
    B. Migraine
    C. Cluster headache
    D. Idiopathic intracranial hypertension

73. A patient presents to the ER with severe throbbing headaches in the right temporal region. There is an association with photophobia, vomiting and sensitivity to sound, along with a history of exacerbation of pain during exertion and relief during sleep. Which of the following diagnoses is most appropriate?

    A. Cluster headaches
    B. Migraine
    C. Idiopathic intracranial hemorrhage
    D. Tension headache

74. A patient presents to the ER with weakness of the leg and urinary and fecal incontinence. Significant findings on examination reveal saddle anesthesia, hypotonia and decreased ankle-jerk reflex. Which of the following diagnoses is most appropriate?

A. Conus medullaris
B. Cauda equina
C. Acute transverse myelitis
D. Lumbar spondylosis

75. A 51-year-old homeless patient is admitted with back pain, which is described as intense and stabbing; urinary incontinence and paresthesia. Significant findings on examination include hypotonia, hyporeflexia and impaired joint position sense of both legs. Also, there is associated ataxia in the heel-shin tests and a positive Romberg sign. Cranial nerve examination reveals Argyll Robertson pupils. Which of the following diagnoses is most likely?

A. Cauda equina
B. Tabes dorsalis
C. Guillain-Barré
D. Poliomyelitis

76. A patient who is being managed for stroke has left hemiparesis and apraxia. Which of the following is most likely the location of the lesion?

A. Cerebellum
B. Hippocampus
C. Thalamus
D. Internal capsule

77. A patient who is being managed for stroke has nystagmus, dysphagia and double vision. In which of these areas is the lesion most likely located?

A. Thalamus
B. Cerebellum
C. Internal capsule
D. Hippocampus

78. A patient presents to the ER with complaints of falling to the ground without any loss of consciousness or confusion. She recalls the event and says this has happened about four times. Which of the following diagnoses is most appropriate?

A. Hypoglycemia
B. Drop attacks
C. Absence seizures
D. Stokes Adams attack

79. A patient who is being managed for stroke has drooping of the left eyelid, with associated miosis and anhidrosis on the left side. Which of the following diagnoses is most accurate?

A. Myasthenia gravis
B. Horner's syndrome
C. Bell's palsy
D. Trigeminal neuralgia

80. A patient presents to the ER with complaints of paroxysmal pain on the left side of her cheek, eyelids and neck. This pain is often triggered by chewing, smiling and brushing of the teeth. Which of the following diagnoses is most appropriate?

A. Trigeminal nerve palsy
B. Bell's palsy
C. Horner's syndrome
D. Trigeminal neuralgia

81. A 45-year-old security officer has nausea, malaise and irritability. Significant findings include a BP of 140/90 mmHg and a history of night-shift work. Which of the following diagnoses is most appropriate?

A. Post-traumatic stress disorder
B. Narcolepsy
C. Insomnia
D. Circadian rhythm disorder

82. A 22-year-old male has excessive daytime sleepiness, cataplexy and hypnagogic hallucinations. Which of the following diagnoses is most appropriate?

    A. Somnambulism
    B. Narcolepsy
    C. Insomnia
    D. Sleep paralysis

83. A 55-year-old smoker is determined to quit smoking with the support of his wife and friends. Which of the following drugs is it inappropriate to prescribe him?

    A. Bupropion
    B. Varenicline
    C. Nicotine
    D. Methadone

84. A patient is worried that she has localized breast cancer. Significant findings include visits to the neighboring hospital for about six months and absent breast masses on palpation. Which of the following diagnoses is most appropriate?

    A. Malingering
    B. Munchausen
    C. Hypochondriasis
    D. Conversion disorder

85. A patient with aplastic anemia complains of severe pain. He is currently on hydrocodone. Which of the following new pain regimens is most appropriate?

    A. Hydromorphone with aspirin
    B. Fentanyl with celecoxib
    C. Hydrocodone with celecoxib
    D. Methadone.

86. A 40-year-old woman with a family history of breast cancer requires mammography for breast cancer screening. Which of the following statements is false?

    A. Mammography should be done yearly.
    B. Mammography should be done every two years.
    C. Mammography should be done every six months.
    D. Mammography should be done every three months.

87. A 22-year-old female with a family history of cervical cancer is about to have a Pap smear for screening. Which of the following statements is correct pertaining to Pap smears?

   A. Screening should be done every two years.
   B. Screening should be done every three years.
   C. Screening should be done monthly.
   D. Screening should be done yearly.

88. A patient being managed for lung carcinoma is admitted with polyphagia, polydipsia and extreme weakness. Significant findings on examination include hyperglycemia, hypokalemia and striae on the abdominal trunk. Which of the following diagnoses is most accurate?

   A. Cushing's disease
   B. Paraneoplastic syndrome
   C. Diabetic ketoacidosis
   D. Tumor lysis syndrome

89. A patient presents to the ER with titubation. Which area of the brain is likely to be affected?

   A. Corpus callosum
   B. Cerebellum
   C. Amygdala
   D. Thalamus

90. A 23-year-old female presents to the ER with painful intercourse, abdominal pain and passage of copious greenish discharge with a fishy odor. Which of the following treatments is most appropriate?

   A. Fluconazole
   B. Metronidazole
   C. Doxycycline
   D. Penicillin

91. A known peptic ulcer disease patient presents to the ER with acute watery diarrhea and abdominal cramps. Significant findings on history and examination reveal recent use of cimetidine and omeprazole. Which of the following interventions is appropriate?

    A. Oral ciprofloxacin
    B. Oral vancomycin
    C. Oral fluconazole
    D. Oral erythromycin

92. A 25-year-old woman presents to the ER with fever, altered sensorium and headaches. She was diagnosed with toxoplasmosis. Which of the following pharmacological interventions is appropriate?

    A. Pyrimethamine
    B. Clindamycin
    C. Pyrimethamine + sulfadiazine
    D. Pyrimethamine + trimethoprim

93. A 20-year-old woman presents to the ER with lower abdominal pain, fever and offensive vaginal discharge. A diagnosis of chlamydia trachomatis is made. Which of the following pharmacological interventions will be most appropriate?

    A. Vancomycin
    B. Doxycycline
    C. Metronidazole
    D. Ciprofloxacin

94. A patient presents to the ER with shortness of breath, dizziness and headaches. BMI is 32 kg/m2. A diagnosis of hypertension is made. Which of the following interventions is not useful for weight reduction?

    A. Substituting water for soft drinks and juices
    B. Avoiding refined carbohydrates and processed food
    C. Bariatric surgery
    D. Limiting calories to at least 55 percent of basal energy expenditure

95. A patient who was recently diagnosed with morbid obesity was placed on orlistat. Which of the following is orlistat's function?

A. An appetite suppressant
B. A 5-HT2C serotonin agonist
C. An inhibitor of intestinal lipase
D. Augments glucose-mediated release from the pancreas

96. A post-op patient complains of shortness of breath. Significant findings on examination include lockjaw, temp 41°C, PR 100 bpm and RR 40 cpm. Which of the following diagnoses is most appropriate?

A. Reactionary hemorrhage
B. Malignant hyperthermia
C. Rhabdomyolysis
D. Hyperkalemia

97. A patient presents to the ER with altered mental status, abnormal motor movement, fast breathing and fever. Significant findings on examination include cogwheel rigidity of the upper limbs, hypertonia, temp 40°C, PPR 120 bpm and RR 40 cpm. The individual is a known psychiatry patient on haloperidol. Which of the following diagnoses is most appropriate?

A. Malignant hyperthermia
B. Delirium tremens
C. Neuroleptic malignant syndrome
D. Serotonin syndrome

98. A patient presents to the ER with agitation, diaphoresis, vomiting and abnormal motor movement. Significant findings on examination include muscular hypertonia, hyperreflexia, spontaneous clonus, temp 39°C, PR 120 bpm and RR 40cpm. The individual is a known psychiatric patient on sertraline. Which of the following diagnoses is most appropriate?

A. Neuroleptic malignant syndrome
B. Serotonin syndrome
C. Malignant hyperthermia
D. Delirium tremens

99. A 24-year-old female presents to the ER with vomiting, altered sensorium, breathlessness and abdominal pain. Significant findings include temp 38°C, RR 40 cpm and PR 120 bpm. A history of aspirin ingestion after a breakup with her boyfriend is obtained. Which of the following interventions is inappropriate?

A. Use of mucomyst
B. Use of activated charcoal
C. Alkaline diuresis
D. Hemodialysis

100. A patient presents to the ER with pain, dizziness and confusion. This patient was brought in by bystanders who claimed he was removed unconscious from his car. Biochemical investigations reveal a carboxyhemoglobin level of 26 percent. Which of the following interventions is most appropriate?

A. Hyperbaric oxygen
B. Red cell transfusion
C. CPAP
D. Surfactant

101. Which of the following poisons is incorrectly matched to its antidote?

A. IV deferoxamine for iron poisoning
B. Dimercaprol for lead poisoning
C. Atropine for organophosphate poisoning
D. Disulfiram for alcohol poisoning

102. A patient presents to the ER with complaints of numbness on the left side of the face. Significant findings on examination include the inability to wrinkle the forehead, blink and grimace. Which of the following diagnoses is most appropriate?

A. Hemispheric stroke
B. Facial nerve palsy
C. Hemifacial spasm
D. Trigeminal neuralgia

103. A patient presents to the ER with paroxysmal attacks of severe pain on the right side of the face when yawning, sneezing and coughing. Which of the following diagnoses is most likely?

A. Bell's palsy
B. Trigeminal neuralgia
C. Herpes simplex
D. Glossopharyngeal neuralgia

104. You are discharging a patient who was recently diagnosed with diabetes mellitus, hypertension and kidney failure. Who should be the primary caretaker of this patient's health-care needs?

A. An endocrinologist
B. A cardiologist
C. A nephrologist
D. A primary health physician

105. Which of the following is the most important outcome of non-adherence?

A. Increased mortality and morbidity
B. Poor patient-nurse relationship
C. Reduced cost of health care
D. Drug-drug interactions

106. Nurse M loves to hand out free drug samples to her patients as an effort to encourage patient adherence. Nurse M must be aware that:

A. Sample drugs are not as effective as the ones sold in the pharmacy.
B. Sample drugs may be cheaper than the ones sold in the pharmacy.
C. Sample drugs do not affect the patient's preference for a particular brand.
D. Sample drugs do not have any marketing goal.

107. A patient with terminal cancer has given an advance directive that forbids all forms of measures except comfort and care. Which of the following principles is being observed?

A. Autonomy
B. Veracity
C. Confidentiality
D. Consent

108. You are providing care to a 17-year-old female who was admitted for attempted suicide. To establish a nurse-patient relationship, which of these actions is necessary?

A. Establish trust by sharing your personal experiences with the patient.
B. Help the patient explore her feelings by giving her a journal and a pen.
C. Talk to the patient as often as you can.
D. Explore your feelings, beliefs and attitudes toward suicide.

109. You are discharging a patient who was admitted for attempted suicide secondary to severe depression. You are to discharge the patient on an MAOI. Which of the following foods is unlikely to cause a hypertensive crisis?

A. Parmesan cheese
B. Salami
C. Tofu
D. Grape juice

110. Which of the following statements is false about the ethical principle of veracity?

A. Health-care workers are expected to be truthful with patients.
B. Health-care workers are expected to honestly share patients' information with their caregivers.
C. Health-care workers are expected to relay information in a way patients can understand.
D. Health-care workers are expected to build a relationship of trust with patients.

111. Nurse J believes that her patient with end-stage bronchial cancer should be baptized by a Roman Catholic priest so his soul will not go to purgatory. Which of the following is being demonstrated?

A. Cultural imposition
B. Cultural conflict
C. Cultural blindness
D. Cultural stereotyping

112. Nurse O says that she does not see why the Jewish patient cannot eat the meat served in the cafeteria like everyone else. Which of the following is being demonstrated?

A. Cultural conflict
B. Cultural blindness
C. Cultural stereotyping
D. Cultural imposition

113. G is a 15-year-old Muslim female from Saudi Arabia who is admitted for severe abdominal pain. Which of the following is correct about obtaining a sexual history from this patient?

    A. It should be obtained in front of the patient's parents.
    B. This history should not be obtained because the patient is not 18.
    C. The history should be obtained in confidence.
    D. This history is not important to the clinical feature.

114. Which of the following questions is most appropriate for obtaining a sexual history from a 16-year-old female who is admitted to the ER with cervicitis

    A. "Do you have a boyfriend?"
    B. "When did you last have sex?"
    C. "What is your sexual orientation?"
    D. "Are you sexually active?"

115. Which of the following is most likely to be seen in a 45-year-old Asian immigrant who was recently diagnosed with stage 3 rectal cancer?

    A. Individuality
    B. Instinct
    C. Communality
    D. Assertion

116. Which of the following questions is most appropriate in obtaining information about sexual orientation from a 25-year-old female who is dressed androgynously?

    A. Are you a lesbian?
    B. Do you consider yourself gay?
    C. Do you sleep with women?
    D. What is your sexual orientation?

117. P is a 45-year-old African American male who is reluctant to partake in a clinical research trial. Which of the following interventions is most appropriate?

    A. Relentlessly provide medical information to ensure he agrees
    B. Tactfully argue the patient out of his reluctance
    C. Accept the patient's wishes
    D. Sign the patient up for the trial without his permission

118. Which of the following approaches is most appropriate in treating a 15-year-old female with a suspected substance abuse disorder?

    A. Order a drug lab test without the patient's consent
    B. Discuss your findings with the patient's parents first
    C. Obtain a drug history of marijuana, alcohol and LSD
    D. Begin with open-ended questions

119. You are about to discharge a patient who was admitted for upper GI bleeding secondary to peptic ulcer disease. Which of the following statements demonstrates the patient's understanding of his condition?

    A. "I should have small, regular meals."
    B. "I should avoid grape juice."
    C. "I should use aspirin for pain."
    D. "Probiotics are useful for lining the ulcers."

120. You are discharging a patient who was admitted for an emergency appendectomy. This patient is not fluent in English. Which of the following interventions is most appropriate?

    A. Write the instructions on paper.
    B. Use flow charts to communicate the instructions.
    C. Play a video for the patient to watch.
    D. Use an interpreter to translate your instructions.

121. You are educating a type 2 diabetic on how to self-administer insulin. Which of the following statements by the patient demonstrates a good grasp of what was taught?

    A. "I should administer the insulin in the same spot every time."
    B. "I should store my insulin in the freezer."
    C. "I should discard used vials every three weeks."
    D. "I should administer insulin in my abdomen."

122. A patient was admitted for cardiac catheterization for myocardial infarction. Which of the following discharge instructions is inappropriate?

    A. Do not lift heavy objects until you are evaluated.
    B. Check your temperature every day for one week.
    C. Drink liberal amounts of water.
    D. Support your head with at least two pillows when sleeping.

123. A patient was admitted for advanced bronchial carcinoma secondary to chronic tobacco use. Which of the following statements demonstrates the patient's understanding of his condition?

    A. "With chemotherapy, I have at least five more years to live."
    B. "A chest X-ray is needed for confirmation."
    C. "I will need to create an advance directive."
    D. "Surgery is curative."

124. You are educating a patient on the proper use of a glucometer. Which of the following statements describes a lack of understanding of the instructions?

    A. "I should use the glucometer before administering insulin."
    B. "I should prick the pad of my finger."
    C. "I should dispose of lancets as soon as they are used."
    D. "I should insert the strip before pricking my finger."

125. Nurse T is presenting her research with the title, "The Challenges of African Americans in Health Care." Which model was used for this research?

    A. Ethnographic model
    B. Phenomenological model
    C. Ground theory mod
    D. Case study model

126. Nurse T is using the descriptive model for research. Which of the following statements is false regarding this model?

    A. It is a model of quantitative research.
    B. It answers the what, how and why of a phenomenon.
    C. It is used to measure data trends.
    D. It can be started without a hypothesis.

127. You have decided to use the quasi-experimental model to conduct your research on opiates and constipation. Which of the following is the key difference between the quasi-experimental model and the experimental model?

    A. In the quasi-experimental model, the independent variable is manipulated.
    B. In the quasi-experimental model, the independent variable is not manipulated.
    C. In the quasi-experimental model, the independent variable is continuous.
    D. In the quasi-experimental model, the independent variable is discrete.

128. You have created a case-control study to investigate tobacco smoking and COPD. Which of the following statements is correct?

   A. Cases are patients with COPD.
   B. Controls will be given tobacco.
   C. Cases will be given tobacco.
   D. Controls are people with COPD.

129. You are conducting a cohort study to assess the effect of a keto diet on patients with diabetes mellitus. Which of the following statements is false?

   A. This is a retrospective observational study.
   B. Subjects in the cohort can be matched.
   C. Cohorts are hard to identify.
   D. The criteria are easy to standardize.

130. You are researching peptic ulcer disease and alcohol consumption. In your sampling method, you divide the members of your population into subgroups of sex and alcohol consumption. What sampling method is this?

   A. Simple sampling
   B. Stratified sampling
   C. Systematic sampling
   D. Clustered sampling

131. Which of the following is not a non-probability sampling method?

   A. Convenience sampling
   B. Snowball sampling
   C. Quota sampling
   D. Clustered sampling

132. Which of the following is not a function of the state Nurse Practice Act?

   A. Setting the standards of requirements for nursing education
   B. Creating reciprocity for licensure among states
   C. Establishing standard salaries for nurses
   D. Maintaining a list of valid nurses in the state

133. An AG-ACNP falsely informs his patient that the nursing assistant attending to him is a lesbian. Which of the following was demonstrated?

A. Slander
B. Libel
C. Gossip
D. Falsehood

134. Which of the following bodies grants the AG-ACNP prescriptive authority?

A. State Nurse Practice Act
B. American Nurses Association
C. State Board of Nursing
D. American Association of Critical-Care Nurses

135. Which of the following is not an element of malpractice?

A. Breach of duty
B. Damage
C. Proximate cause
D. Impairment

136. An AG-ACNP performs a venipuncture on a patient without seeking informed consent. Which of the following is demonstrated?

A. Assault
B. Battery
C. Malpractice
D. Negligence

137. As an AG-ACNP, you suspect a registered nurse on your team is suffering from impairment caused by alcohol intoxication. Which of the following steps is most appropriate?

A. Confirm your suspicion from the nurses' colleagues
B. Request a blood alcohol test
C. Send the nurse to a psychiatrist for evaluation
D. Suspend the nurse

138. An AG-ACNP discusses the condition of one of her patients with her friend. Which of the following has been breached?

  A. Fidelity
  B. Justice
  C. Confidentiality
  D. Beneficence

139. Which of the following interventions is inappropriate for a patient who just had an external fixation for an open fracture of the right tibia?

  A. Provide a fracture pan.
  B. Encourage isometric exercises
  C. Provide a high-protein diet
  D. Perform routine enemas

140. Which of the following interventions is inappropriate for a 45-year-old patient with emphysema whose BMI is 17.5 kg/m2?

  A. Give high-calorie foods in larger quantities.
  B. Avoid carbonated beverages.
  C. Increase fluid intake.
  D. Administer oxygen during meals via nasal prongs.

141. A 55-year-old male with chronic bronchitis complains of shortness of breath even while on oxygen. Important findings on examination include flaring of the nasal alar and tachypnea. Which of the following interventions is inappropriate in providing basic care and comfort?

  A. Splint the chest wall with a pillow.
  B. Suction the airway.
  C. Give cromoglycate.
  D. Inspect the oxygen delivery system.

142. A morbidly obese patient just had gastric bypass surgery. Which of the following interventions is inappropriate in reducing the risk of deep vein thrombosis?

  A. Inspect the calf for a positive Homan's sign.
  B. Provide Gingko biloba supplements.
  C. Provide prophylactic heparin.
  D. Use compression stockings.

143. A patient with left ventricular heart failure has a temperature of 38°C. Significant findings on examination include chills and rigors. Which of the following interventions is not appropriate?

    A. Provide IV antipyretics.
    B. Adjust the environmental temperature.
    C. Provide IV diazepam.
    D. Provide IV hydrocortisone.

144. A patient who has just had an emergency appendectomy complains of pain. Which of the following interventions is inappropriate in reducing the risk of post-op pain?

    A. Put the patient in the semi-Fowler's position.
    B. Place the patient on NPO.
    C. Place the patient in the supine position.
    D. Give the patient analgesia as needed.

145. A patient has just had an emergency cholecystectomy. Which of the following will not reduce the risk of skin breakdown?

    A. Changing the wound dressing as often as indicated
    B. Assessing the incisional tubes for kinks
    C. Monitoring the sclera for jaundice
    D. Place the patient in the supine position

146. You are the newly elected nursing representative of the disciplinary committee. Which of the following techniques is most appropriate in resolving conflicts?

    A. Avoidance
    B. Tolerance
    C. Compromise
    D. Aggressiveness

147. You are reviewing the job applications of registered nurses applying to the hospital. One of these nurses has a functional impairment of her left leg. However, she has the right to employment because:

    A. She is a member of the American Nurses Association.
    B. Her impairment is not cognitive.
    C. She is a citizen of the United States.
    D. She is protected by the Americans with Disabilities Act.

148. As the head of your health team, you are responsible for providing a performance appraisal for all your team members. Which of the following principles is incorrect?

A. Verbal appraisals are more useful than written appraisals.
B. Patients are subjective assessments of a team member's performance.
C. Performance appraisals should focus on areas of strengths and weaknesses.
D. Performance appraisals should be focused on improving performance.

149. Nurse M is a nursing unit head who is fond of conducting spontaneous, informal appraisals. Which of the following is a disadvantage of such an approach?

A. It creates room for confrontation and collaboration.
B. Subjective data is collected.
C. It is natural.
D. It can provide insight when compiling a formal report.

150. On Nurse T's team, all members of the team report to her directly and consult her for any action that is to be taken. What form of organizational structure is this?

A. Centralized
B. Decentralized
C. Matrix
D. Authoritarian

Test 3: Answers and Explanations

1. (D) Flattened hemi-diaphragms.

The following are chest X-ray findings of heart failure: an enlarged cardiac silhouette, Kerley B lines and pleural effusion, which causes blunting of the costophrenic angle. Flattened hemi-diaphragms are typically seen in hyperinflated lungs.

2. (A) Increased capillary hydrostatic pressure.

This patient has pleural effusion that is caused by increased capillary hydrostatic pressure secondary to left ventricular heart failure.

3. (C) Beta-blockers.

Beta-blockers are contraindicated in patients with diastolic heart failure because lowering their heart rate can exacerbate symptoms. This is because patients with diastolic heart failure have a relatively fixed stroke volume, which makes their cardiac output heart rate–dependent.

4. (D) Prompt commencement of chest physiotherapy is called for.

Patients with prosthetic valves are at increased risk of infective endocarditis and thromboembolic episodes. When placed on anticoagulation therapies, they are at risk for bleeding disorders. Complications of prosthetic valves also include pulmonary hypertension, valve rejection and others. Chest physiotherapy is not indicated.

5. (C) Atenolol.

Beta-blockers like atenolol are suitable for treating sinus tachycardia. Enalapril and Losartan are unsuitable because the patient has no other complications. Digoxin is unsuitable because it shortens refractoriness.

6. (C) Tension pneumothorax.

Although tension pneumothorax, hemothorax and cardiac tamponade present with similar features, tension pneumothorax presents with unilateral absent breath sounds and hyperresonant notes on the affected side.

7. (C) Tricuspid regurgitation.

Features of tricuspid regurgitation include recurrent breathlessness, a holosystolic murmur and features of right ventricular failure.

8. (B) Pulmonary embolism.

This patient is obese and is therefore at risk for deep vein thrombosis and consequent pulmonary embolism.

9. (C) Percutaneous angiography.

This patient has an NSTEMI. Although oxygen administration, thrombolytics and anticoagulants are necessary, they are all part of supportive management. Definite treatment is percutaneous angiography.

10. (B) 0.9% saline.

To reduce the risk of contrast nephropathy, proper hydration is necessary. This is done with 0.9% saline given at 1 ml/kg 24 hours before the procedure.

11. (C) Ionic contrast agents are hypoosmolar to the blood.

This treatment is incorrect because ionic agents are hyperosmolar to the blood and increase the risk for neurotoxicity and pulmonary edema.

12. (C) Amlodipine.

Amlodipine is a calcium channel blocker and is an ideal hypertensive to administer in this situation. Black individuals and people of African descent respond better to calcium channel blockers and diuretics.

13. (B) Unstable angina.

The features of unstable angina include chest pain that occurs at rest and lasts more than twenty minutes. This chest pain may be accompanied by dyspnea and diaphoresis. Also, angina increases in intensity and duration and lowers in the threshold.

14. (D) 24-hour BP monitoring.

This patient most likely has orthostatic hypotension that is caused by her blood pressure drugs. Antihypertensives like calcium channel blockers, ACE inhibitors and nitroglycerin can cause postural hypotension.

15. (B) Hypertrophic cardiomyopathy.

This is the most common cause of death in young athletes. Other causes include commotio cordis, anomalies of the coronary arteries, myocarditis, ruptured aortic aneurysms and others.

16. (B) Lisinopril.

ACE inhibitors and ARBs are ideal for Caucasians. They are also renoprotective.

17. (B) Hypertensive kidney disease.

Chronic and uncontrolled hypertension can cause hypertensive kidney disease. Bilaterally shrunken kidneys are typically found in such cases.

18. (A) Labetalol.

In this patient, the blood pressure should be brought down gradually using an intravenous, titratable antihypertensive, like nitroprusside, fenoldopam, nicardipine, labetalol or hydralazine. Oral drugs are not useful, and antihypertensives that crash the blood pressure should be avoided.

19. (B) Stop spironolactone.

Gynecomastia is a side effect of spironolactone, an aldosterone antagonist. The appropriate intervention is to stop spironolactone.

20. (B) Stop spironolactone.

This patient has hyperkalemia. Spironolactone is a potassium-sparing diuretic and should be stopped. Although hemodialysis is used for hyperkalemia, the indication is serum potassium that is greater than 6 mmol/L.

21. (A) Supine position.

To avoid maneuvering the neck, the patient is placed flat in the supine position. The chin lift or jaw-thrust maneuver is then used to assess the airway. The sniffling position is contraindicated for patients with a suspected cervical injury.

22. (B) Emergency bronchoscopy.

This patient has an airway obstruction caused by an airway tumor. An emergency bronchoscopy will provide relief from the obstructed airway and allow specimens to be taken for histology.

23. (C) Bronchiectasis.

The patient has clinical features and chest X-ray findings that are in keeping with bronchiectasis.

24. (A) Deterioration of clinical symptoms lasting for at least 48 hours.

An exacerbation of bronchiectasis is defined as deterioration for at least 48 hours in ≥ 3 of the following: cough, sputum purulence, sputum volume, shortness of breath, fatigue and hemoptysis.

25. (D) Pulmonary vascular hypertrophy.

Primary pulmonary hypertension is caused by an increase in the vascular resistance of either/both pulmonary veins and arteries. This is usually triggered by obliteration of the vascular beds with or without pathologic vasoconstriction. Option A describes cor pulmonale; option B describes Eisenmenger's syndrome and option C describes COPD.

26. (A) Pulmonary vasodilators.

Pulmonary vasodilators like hydralazine, calcium channel blockers and nitrous oxide are effective only for patients with primary pulmonary hypertension.

27. (B) A chest X-ray is likely to show subpleural reticular opacities.

This statement is false because the clinical examination of the chest shows lobar involvement on the right hemithorax. Lobar infiltration is most likely to be seen on a chest X-ray.

28. (C) Moraxella catarrhalis.

This is a gram-negative diplococcus that is implicated in community-acquired pneumonia.

29. (B) Ventilator-associated pneumonia.

Ventilator-associated pneumonia develops in a patient at least 48 hours after endotracheal intubation.

30. (A) Positioning the patient in the recumbent position.

The recumbent position increases the risk of infection. To reduce the risk of pneumonia, the patient is placed in the high Fowler's or semi-Fowler's position.

31. (D) Trimethoprim/sulfamethoxazole.

This patient most likely has pneumonia caused by pneumocystis jirovecii. Treatment is with trimethoprim/sulfamethoxazole.

32. (D) Blood culture.

This patient has pulmonary tuberculosis. A blood culture is not appropriate for diagnosis. Diagnosis is made from the clinical history, chest X-ray, acid-fast stain, anti-tuberculin skin test and nucleic acid-based test.

33. (C) Ethambutol.

Optic neuritis is an adverse effect of ethambutol, especially when it is given at high doses. Symptoms are usually reversible on early detection. Patients are advised to have regular visual acuity and color vision testing.

34. (B) Chronic bronchitis.

The key features of chronic bronchitis are progressive breathlessness, wheezing and a cough that is productive of sputum, although not as copious as that of bronchiectasis. Also, the FEV1/FVC ratio before bronchodilation is 64 percent, which improves to 65 percent after administering bronchodilators.

35. (A) Noninvasive positive pressure ventilation.

Noninvasive positive pressure ventilation is indicated for patients who do not respond to pharmacological interventions. In this patient, mechanical ventilation should be performed immediately.

36. (B) Pleural biopsy.

This patient has a significant history of asbestos exposure. The best investigation to confirm mesothelioma is a pleural biopsy.

37. (B) Empyema.

This patient most likely has a lung abscess from aspiration of infected oral secretions. Her social status as a homeless person and the presence of poor oral hygiene are features that point to the diagnosis.

38. (A) Hyponatremia.

These patients have hyponatremia caused by polydipsia and enhanced secretion of vasopressin.

39. (A) Serum T3 is very sensitive for screening.

This statement is false. Serum TSH is the most sensitive test for diagnosing hypothyroidism. Because patients with primary hypothyroidism have normal circulating levels of T3 from persistent TSH secretion, serum T3 screening is not sensitive.

40. (C) Propylthiouracil.

This drug is preferable for treatment because the dosages partially block the peripheral conversion of T4 to T3.

41. (C) Exophthalmos.

Clinical features that do not respond to beta-blockers include goiter, bruit, exophthalmos, weight loss, increased oxygen consumption and increased circulating thyroxine levels.

42. (D) Methimazole is readily converted to carbimazole.

This statement is false because carbimazole is converted to methimazole.

43. (D) Thyrotoxicosis.

Thyrotoxicosis is a life-threatening exacerbation of hyperthyroidism. Patients are typically ineligible for surgery until their thyroid levels are stabilized.

44. (B) Polycythemia rubra.

The key features of polycythemia rubra are hyperviscosity syndrome (weakness, headaches, visual disturbances, aquagenic pruritus and shortness of breath), splenomegaly and an elevated red blood cell count that is greater than 16 g/dL.

45. (B) Blast cells.

This patient most likely has leukemia (AML). Diagnosis is confirmed when the myeloid blast cells are 20 percent or more of nonerythroid cells.

46. (C) Hepatomegaly.

Hepatomegaly is an unusual feature of Hodgkin's lymphoma. Splenomegaly is typically present.

47. (B) Protein electrophoresis.

The diagnosis of multiple myeloma involves the demonstration of M proteins in the serum and the presence of excessive plasma cells in the bone marrow. The other listed investigations are supportive.

48. (D) Ferroportin disease.

Ferroportin disease is a type of primary (not secondary) hemochromatosis. It is also called Type 4 hereditary hemochromatosis.

49. (A) Massive transfusion.

Fresh-frozen plasma and platelets are used for massive blood transfusion to reduce the risk of dilutional thrombocytopenia. Massive transfusion does not indicate cryoprecipitate transfusion.

50. (A) TIPS procedure.

TIPS (transjugular intrahepatic portosystemic shunt) is a procedure used for persistent and/or recurring bleeds. It is an emergency technique that shunts blood from the portal circulation into the IVC, lowers portal pressure and reduces bleeding.

Mechanical compression of bleeding varices with a Sengstaken-Blakemore tube increases mortality and should not be used as primary management. Liver transplantation can decompress the portal system, but it is only useful to patients on a transplant list.

51. (C) Providing a protein-free diet.

This measure will not be useful because patients with decompensated liver failure are likely to be malnourished. Rather than cut down on protein, vegetable protein is used as the primary protein source.

52. (B) Bilirubin is excreted in the urine.

Option A is false because hepatitis is a form of conjugated hyperbilirubinemia. As such, bilirubin will be excreted in the urine. Option C is incorrect because jaundice occurs when serum bilirubin is 33 to 51 umol/L. Option D is false because pruritus is a usual feature due to deposition of bile salts in the epidermis.

53. (A) Relaxation of the lower esophageal sphincter.

Acid reflux occurs when there is a reflux of gastric contents into the esophagus. This reflux is caused by a relaxed/incompetent lower esophageal sphincter. Option B describes a hiatal hernia; option C describes an esophageal web and option D describes achalasia.

54. (C) Loperamide.

This drug is an antimotility agent and is therefore inappropriate. Antimotility agents are contraindicated in patients with bloody diarrhea because of suspected E. coli infection.

55. (B) IBS.

This patient has features of irritable bowel syndrome, which is characterized by recurrent abdominal discomfort that either occurs with defecation, with a change in frequency of stool or with a change in the consistency of stool.

56. (D) Use of hypertonic 3% saline.

Hypertonic saline is useful for patients with severe hyponatremia and rapid onset hyponatremia. However, this fluid increases the risk of osmotic demyelination syndrome. Therefore, aggressive sodium correction should be done judiciously.

57. (D) Central diabetes insipidus.

Central diabetes insipidus is a cause of euvolemic hyponatremia, whereby there is a decrease in total body water with almost normal total body sodium.

58. (C) Prophylactic antibiotics.

Prophylactic antibiotics are not useful for patients who require long-term catheterization.

59. (C) Candida.

This patient has cervicitis that is being demonstrated by a positive cervical motion tenderness. Candida is not the usual cause of cervicitis.

60. (B) Bladder cancer.

Painless hematuria is a usual finding in bladder cancer. It is usually accompanied by irritative urinary tract symptoms, symptoms of anemia, pelvic pain and palpable masses in the suprapubic region. This patient's occupational history in the textile industry places him at risk for bladder cancer due to chronic exposure to aromatic compounds in the dye.

61. (D) Retrograde urethrography.

This patient has acute urinary retention caused by a urethral stricture. Clinical diagnosis is made based on age and difficulty in passing the urethral catheter. Definitive diagnosis is confirmed by a retrograde urethrography or cystoscopy.

62. (C) Testicular torsion.

This patient has testicular torsion. The classic features of testicular torsion include severe scrotal pain, nausea, vomiting, fever and urinary frequency. On examination, there is edema and induration of the affected scrotum. Cremasteric reflex is absent, and the testes are elevated and horizontal.

63. (A) Herniorrhaphy.

This patient has a strangulated inguinal hernia that requires an urgent excision of the inguinal sac and repair of the posterior wall. Herniotomy is inappropriate here because it only involves excision of the inguinal sac; this is commonly done in pediatric patients.

64. (B) Bullous pemphigoid.

The features in this history that support this diagnosis include age that is greater than 60, fluid vesicles that are on the flexure areas of the upper and lower limbs, negative Nikolsky sign and lesions that spare the mucocutaneous surfaces.

65. (C) Cellulitis.

Significant aspects of this history that support this diagnosis include unilateral tenderness of the left leg, erythema, warmth and peau d' orange.

66. (D) Autoimmune reaction.

This patient has psoriasis, a skin disorder that is characterized by rapid cell turnover. Although the exact cause of psoriasis remains unknown, it is believed to be triggered by a combination of environmental and genetic factors. It can be caused by autoimmune reactions to skin cells. Psoriasis runs in families.

67. (B) Ankylosing spondylitis.

This patient has the classic features of ankylosing spondylitis, a systemic disorder that causes inflammation of the axial skeleton and large peripheral joints. Symptoms include nocturnal back pain, back stiffness and kyphosis, reduced chest expansion and constitutional symptoms.

68. (B) Psoriatic arthritis.

This patient has the classic features of psoriatic arthritis, which includes psoriasis of the skin and asymmetric arthritis of the upper and lower limbs, the most common joints being the DIP joint of the fingers and toes.

69. (B) Celecoxib.

Although NSAIDs are used in the management of rheumatoid arthritis, they are not classified as disease-modifying antirheumatic drugs because they do not slow down the progression of rheumatoid arthritis.

70. (A) Order a serum creatinine kinase assay.

This patient has rhabdomyolysis from a crush injury. Diagnosis is made from serum creatine kinase levels that are five times the upper limit of normal. An emergency fasciotomy is not appropriate because nothing in the patient's history shows an underlying compartment syndrome.

71. (B) Giant cell arteritis.

This patient has the classic features of arteritis, which include headache in the temporal region; prominent temporal arteritis, which may have nodules or erythema on the overlying skin; visual disturbances and unexplained anemia or fever. Diagnostic tests reveal elevated C-reactive protein and ESR. Diagnosis is confirmed by biopsy of the temporal arteries.

72. (C) Cluster headache.

The distinct features of cluster headache are unilateral and very painful headaches that occur in the orbitotemporal region. These headaches peak and subside spontaneously in about 30 to 60 minutes. There are associated with autonomic features, like rhinorrhea, lacrimation, facial flushing and Horner's syndrome. Unlike migraine headaches, patients with cluster headaches are restless and agitated.

73. (B) Migraine.

The classic features of a migraine include severe and throbbing unilateral headaches that are associated with nausea and sensitivity to light, sound or odors. Headaches are usually exacerbated by exertion and relieved by sleep. Patients also complain of auras that occur just before the headache starts.

74. (B) Cauda equina.

In cauda equina syndrome, there is distal leg paresis, saddle anesthesia (sensory loss in and around the perineum and anus) and dysfunction of the bladder and anus. Although symptoms match those of conus medullaris, there is decreased muscle tone and slow deep tendon reflex in the legs.

75. (B) Tabes dorsalis.

Features of tabes dorsalis include intense stabbing pain in the back and legs, gait ataxia, hyperesthesia, paresthesia and loss of sensation to the bladder. Patients with tabes dorsalis have sad facies, Argyll Robertson pupils and optic atrophy. Examination of the legs reveals hypotonia, hyporeflexia, impaired vibratory and joint position sense, ataxia and a positive Romberg sign.

76. (D) Internal capsule.

Lesions in the internal capsule are characterized by hemiparesis and apraxia. Lesions in the hippocampus cause memory loss. Lesions in the cerebellum cause movement and balance disorders. Lesions in the thalamus cause disorders of arousal, orientation, learning, memory and other aspects of cognition.

77. (B) Cerebellum.

Lesions in the cerebellum are characterized by unilateral or bilateral cranial nerve deficits that cause nystagmus, vertigo, dysphagia, dysarthria, diplopia and blindness. Other features include limb ataxia, spastic paresis, labile blood pressure and cardiopulmonary arrest. Lesions in the thalamus cause disorders of arousal, orientation, learning, memory and other aspects of cognition. Lesions in the internal capsule are characterized by hemiparesis and apraxia. Lesions in the hippocampus cause memory loss.

78. (B) Drop attacks.

Drop attacks are characterized by spontaneous falls while a patient is standing or walking. There is no loss of consciousness or amnesia.

79. (B) Horner's syndrome.

The classic features of Horner's syndrome include ptosis, miosis, hyperemia and anhidrosis on the affected side of the face.

80. (D) Trigeminal neuralgia.

Features of trigeminal neuralgia include severe pain on the affected side of the face that is supplied by the trigeminal nerve. This pain is often paroxysmal and triggered by smiling, brushing or chewing.

81. (D) Circadian rhythm disorder.

In this disorder, the sleep-wake cycle and the external day and night cycle are desynchronized. The causes may be internal, such as advanced sleep phase syndrome, or external, like shift work. In this patient, frequent rotation of his night shift has affected his sleep-wake cycle.

82. (B) Narcolepsy.

The main features of narcolepsy include excessive daytime sleepiness, cataplexy, hypnagogic and hypnagogic hallucinations, sleep paralysis and disturbed nocturnal sleep.

83. (D) Methadone.

Methadone is an opioid agonist-antagonist used for patients with opioid addiction. It is not appropriate to help people quit smoking.

84. (C) Hypochondriasis.

This patient has the classic features of hypochondriasis/illness anxiety disorder, which includes preoccupation with an illness for more than six months with minimal or absent somatic symptoms, repeated visits to the hospital or a maladaptive avoidance of hospital and doctor appointments. Symptoms are usually not attributed to depression or other mental health disorders.

85. (D) Methadone.

This option is most appropriate because methadone is suitable for severe chronic pain caused by incurable diseases, like cancer. Most importantly, the use of NSAIDs and aspirin is contraindicated in patients with aplastic anemia because of the risk of bleeding.

86. (A) Mammography should be done yearly.

The American Cancer Society recommends that women ages 40 to 44 and 45 to 54 should have yearly mammograms as long as they are in good health.

87. (B) Screening should be done every three years.

According to the American Cancer Society, a Pap smear should be done every three years for women between ages 21 and 29.

88. (B) Paraneoplastic syndrome.

This patient has Cushing syndrome that is characterized by high cortisol, which causes hyperglycemia, hypokalemia and truncal obesity. Option B is correct because in this case, the excess cortisol is released as a result of the lung carcinoma secreting ACTH/ACTH molecules.

89. (B) Cerebellum.

Titubation, which is shaking/nodding of the head or body, is a sign of cerebellar disease.

90. (B) Metronidazole.

This patient has trichomoniasis, a sexually transmitted infection caused by the flagellated protozoan Trichomonas vaginalis. Treatment includes metronidazole therapy for both the patient and her sexual partner(s).

91. (B) Oral vancomycin.

This patient most likely has gastroenteritis caused by clostridium difficile. Risk factors for infection with clostridium difficile include extreme age, prolonged hospitalization, chronic use of antibiotics and use of proton pump inhibitors and H2 receptor blockers.

92. (C) Pyrimethamine + sulfadiazine.

This woman is immunocompromised and has CNS toxoplasmosis. The treatment regimen is pyrimethamine + sulfadiazine.

93. (B) Doxycycline.

The treatment of uncomplicated chlamydia trachomatis includes a single dose of azithromycin or doxycycline given twice daily for seven days; erythromycin given for seven days or ofloxacin or levofloxacin, each given for seven days.

94. (D) Limiting calories to at least 55 percent of basal energy expenditure.

This intervention is inappropriate because a very low-calorie diet is unlikely to yield results on a long-term basis.

95. (C) An inhibitor of intestinal lipase.

Orlistat inhibits intestinal lipase, decreases fat absorption and improves serum glucose and lipid levels. Side effects include flatus, the passage of bulky and oily stools and diarrhea. Option A is the mechanism of action of phentermine. Option B is the mechanism of action of Lorcaserin, and option D is the mechanism of action of Liraglutide.

96. (B) Malignant hyperthermia.

Malignant hyperthermia occurs during anesthesia (succinylcholine and halothane) or in the early postoperative period. Clinical features include muscle rigidity in the jaw, tachycardia, tachypnea, arrhythmia, hypercapnia and hyperpyrexia.

97. (C) Neuroleptic malignant syndrome.

The clinical features of neuroleptic malignant syndrome include altered mental status, motor abnormalities, hyperpyrexia and increased autonomic activity. Causes include the use of drugs like first-generation antipsychotics like haloperidol, chlorpromazine and loxapine, and other newer antipsychotics, like clozapine, olanzapine, risperidone and others.

98. (B) Serotonin syndrome.

The classic features of serotonin syndrome include muscle hypertonia, spontaneous clonus, tremor, hyperreflexia, diaphoresis, hyperpyrexia and ocular or inducible clonus. There is usually a history of serotonergic drugs that are taken either as self-poisoning or therapeutically.

99. (A) Use of mucomyst.

This intervention is inappropriate because mucomyst is used for acetaminophen poisoning. Mucomyst (N-acetylcysteine) is a precursor of glutathione that increases the hepatic stores of glutathione. It reduces the rate of hepatotoxicity by binding to acetaminophen metabolite before it destroys the hepatocytes.

100. (A) Hyperbaric oxygen.

This patient has carbon monoxide poisoning, probably obtained from his automobile. Because his carboxyhemoglobin level is > 25%, this patient will benefit from hyperbaric oxygen. The indications for hyperbaric oxygen include cardiopulmonary instability, altered sensorium, loss of consciousness and a carboxyhemoglobin level that is greater than 25%.

101. (D) Disulfiram for alcohol poisoning.

Disulfiram is incorrectly matched to its antidote. It is used for alcoholics who are willing to overcome their drinking habits. It is not used for alcohol intoxication. Management principles for alcohol intoxication include IV glucose, IV fluids, correction of electrolyte imbalance and use of IV proton pump inhibitors.

102. (B) Facial nerve palsy.

The features of facial nerve palsy include weakness and numbness on the affected side and an inability to wrinkle the forehead, blink or grimace. In more severe cases, there is a widening of the palpebral fissure, which can irritate the conjunctiva.

103. (D) Glossopharyngeal neuralgia.

Glossopharyngeal neuralgia is characterized by excruciating pain that is unilateral and paroxysmal. Pain occurs when the patient is yawning, coughing, sneezing, swallowing or talking, or when using any muscle that is innervated by the glossopharyngeal nerve. The pain typically begins in the tonsillar region or at the base of the ear and spreads to the ear of the affected area.

104. (D) A primary health physician.

The primary health physician is the primary provider of this patient's needs. The primary health physician must refer her to the endocrinologist, cardiologist and nephrologist when the need arises.

105. (A) Increased mortality and morbidity.

This is the most significant outcome in patient non-adherence to drugs and treatment. Non-adherence can lead to microbial resistance, as in the case of antibiotics therapy; worsening clinical conditions; increased stress on the immune system and death.

106. (B) Sample drugs may be cheaper than the ones sold in the pharmacy.

Part of the marketing strategies for drug representatives is to give discounted drug samples. These samples do not give a clear insight into the cost of their generic counterparts in the market. Option A is incorrect because sample drugs are just as effective as the ones in the pharmacy. Options C and D are incorrect because sample drugs are part of the marketing goals of drug reps, and they do influence a patient's preference for a particular brand.

107. (A) Autonomy.

In ethics, autonomy is the principle that states that patients have a right to refuse or accept medical treatment based on their preferences and without coercion.

108. (D) Explore your feelings, beliefs and attitudes towards suicide.

This step, which is known as the orientation phase, helps the nurse practitioner discover his or her personal attitudes and perceptions. The nurse must be self-aware before attempting to establish a relationship with the patient.

109. (D) Grape juice.

Grape juice is unlikely to cause a hypertensive crisis. Hypertensive crises can arise when tyramine-rich foods are consumed along with MAOIs. Foods that are rich in tyramine include foods that are aged, cured, pickled or fermented. Examples include aged cheeses like parmesan, American, ricotta and cottage cheeses; cured meats like pepperoni, sausage, salami, corned beef and others; pickled foods like kimchi, tofu and pickles; and fermented wines and beers.

110. (B) Health workers are expected to honestly share patients' information with the caregiver.

This statement is false because it violates the principle of confidentiality. Health workers are only allowed to divulge information that has been consented to by the patient.

111. (A) Cultural imposition.

This occurs when health workers think that their values, beliefs and practices are superior to a patient's and then attempt to impose such on the patient.

112. (B) Cultural blindness.

This occurs when a person treats everyone the same without noticing the cultural differences that exist among people.

113. (C) The history should be obtained in confidence.

Option A is incorrect because it violates the principle of confidentiality. Options B and C are incorrect because the history is significant to the clinical feature and, therefore, must be obtained for proper clinical management.

114. (D) "Are you sexually active?"

This statement is most appropriate because it is formal and professional. Options A and B are incorrect because they are assuming and prejudiced. Option C is incorrect because the aim is to confirm a history of sexual activity regardless of sexual orientation.

115. (C) Communality.

The Asian immigrant is most likely to demonstrate communality and communal dependence on members of his family in terms of social support and decision-making. Kinship is a common feature demonstrated among people from Asia.

116. (D) What is your sexual orientation?

This approach is most appropriate because it is formal, professional and free from bias. All the other options are based on assumptions that can offend the patient.

117. (C) Accept the patient's wishes.

This is the most appropriate response because it obeys the principle of informed consent and the principles of autonomy, beneficence and confidentiality in ethics.

118. (D) Begin with open-ended questions.

This is the most appropriate approach because it is professional, formal and unbiased. Other options are not only unprofessional but violate the principles of confidentiality.

119. (A) "I should have small, regular meals."

Small, regular meals reduce the occurrence of bloating and dyspepsia, satiety and indigestion. Option B is incorrect because grape juice does not increase hyperacidity. Option C is incorrect because aspirin and NSAIDs are generally avoided as they erode the gastric mucosa. Option D is incorrect because probiotics have not been shown to treat PUD.

120. (D) Use an interpreter to translate your instructions.

This is the most appropriate response to ensure that the patient understands what is being said. Options A, B and C are all inappropriate because you cannot objectively assess the patient's understanding of the information conveyed.

121. (D) "I should administer insulin in my abdomen."

The abdomen is the most preferred location for insulin injections because of its wide surface area. It can also hide features of lipohypertrophy. Option A is incorrect because administering insulin in the same site increases the risk of lipohypertrophy. Option B is incorrect because insulin should never be stored at extreme temperatures. Option C is incorrect because used vials are viable for a month.

122. (D) Support your head with at least two pillows when sleeping.

This statement is inappropriate because it will not help promote the patient's recovery. The patient may sleep with a pillow to relieve the symptoms of orthopnea if he is in heart failure.

123. (C) "I will need to create an advance directive."

This statement is accurate because patients with advanced bronchogenic carcinoma have less than a 1 percent chance of living for five years. Lung cancer has the highest mortality rate in the United States. Confirmation is done by biopsy. Surgery and chemotherapy are not curative.

124. (B) "I should prick the pad of my finger."

This statement is false because the pads of the fingers are generally avoided as they are more painful. Also, calluses formed on the pads of the fingers can interfere with biometric tests.

125. (B) Phenomenological model.

The phenomenological model involves the use of surveys, questionnaires and interviews that describe how a participant experiences an event.

126. (B) It answers the what, how and why of a phenomenon.

This statement is false because descriptive research attempts to describe the characteristics of a phenomenon—that is the what, how, where and when. It does not attempt to answer why. This research aims to understand the attributes and characteristics of a phenomenon before going on to explain the reason for its existence. This is why the research can be started without a hypothesis.

127. (B) In the quasi-experimental model, the independent variable is not manipulated.

Unlike the true experimental model, in which the independent variable is manipulated to establish the cause-effect relationship between two variables; in the quasi-experimental model, the independent variable is not manipulated and the researcher uses pre-existing groups.

128. (A) Cases are patients with COPD.

A case study compares patients who have a disease with subjects who do not have the disease. It is a retrospective study that observes how the frequency of exposure to a risk factor determines the causal effect. In this example, the case study is patients who smoked tobacco and have COPD, while the control group is subjects who also smoke tobacco but do not have COPD.

129. (A) This is a retrospective observational study.

This statement is false because a cohort study is a prospective observational study in which samples/cohorts are followed in a chronological manner, and evaluations are made on a disease outcome.

130. (B) Stratified sampling.

In the stratified sampling method, the sampling population is divided into subgroups of people who share a similar characteristic. This method is used when the researcher expects to see variability between the subgroups and wants to ensure that each subgroup is properly represented.

131. (D) Clustered sampling.

This is not a non-probability sampling method. Non-probability sampling methods include convenience sampling, snowball sampling, quota sampling, purposive sampling and bias-in sampling. Probability sampling methods include stratified sampling, clustered sampling, systematic sampling and simple random sampling.

132. (C) Establishing the standard salary for nurses.

The State Nurse Practice Act is not responsible for establishing standard nurses' salaries. Negotiation for remuneration is between the nurses and their representatives from a union or financial organization and their employers.

133. (A) Slander.

Slander is a form of defamation in which the perpetrator issues a false statement to discredit someone's character or nature. Slander is spoken, while libel is written and published either online or in print.

134. (A) State Nurse Practice Act.

The State Nurse Practice Act is responsible for establishing the standard of nursing practice in the state. One of these standards involves granting nursing practitioners prescriptive rights according to state law.

135. (D) Impairment.

Impairment is not an element of malpractice. The four elements include the nurse's duty to the patient; a breach of duty; proximate cause, which means the occurrence of injury from the breach of duty; and damage, which is the relationship between the injury and the nurse's breach of duty.

136. (B) Battery.

In nursing practice, battery occurs when the nurse touches a patient without obtaining consent. Battery is an intentional tort covered under civil law.

137. (B) Request a blood alcohol level test.

This step is most appropriate because it is objective and non-assuming. It is difficult to get an objective response from the nurse's colleagues, and it is inappropriate to take further actions without due verification.

138. (C) Confidentiality.

This nurse has breached the ethical principle of confidentiality. Confidentiality means that a patient's health information is accessible only by authorized personnel. Fidelity is the ability of a nurse to keep to a promise.

139. (D) Perform routine enemas.

This intervention is inappropriate because enemas are not done routinely. Although this patient is at risk of having constipation (caused by use of analgesic and immobility), measures to reduce the risk of constipation include early ambulation, increase of fluid intake and provision of a high-fiber diet.

140. (A) Give high-calorie foods in larger quantities.

This intervention is inappropriate because high-calorie foods should be given in smaller portions. Patients with emphysema are often anorexic, so offering foods in larger quantities will discourage them from eating.

141. (C) Give cromoglycate.

This intervention is inappropriate because cromoglycate is a mast cell stabilizer used to reduce the incidence of IgE-mediated asthmatic attacks. Although this patient has an obstructive airway disease, chronic bronchitis is caused by remodeling of the airway due to chronic inflammation of the bronchioles and not by an allergic hyperactive airway.

142. (B) Provide Gingko biloba supplements.

This intervention is inappropriate because Gingko biloba has the potential of interacting with the prescribed anticoagulant, thereby reducing its therapeutic index. Gingko biloba increases the patient's risk of developing a DVT.

143. (D) Provide IV hydrocortisone.

This patient most likely has pneumonia caused by pulmonary congestion. Interventions should be aimed at controlling the fever, improving oxygenation and tissue perfusion and commencing intravenous antibiotics. IV hydrocortisone will not be useful to this patient.

144. (C) Place the patient in the supine position.

This intervention is inappropriate because, in the supine position, the inflammatory exudates do not gravitate toward the lower abdomen or pelvis. This can cause tension in the abdomen and pain.

145. (D) Place the patient in the supine position.

This intervention is inappropriate because the patient is placed in the low or semi-Fowler's position to encourage gravitational drainage of bile.

146. (C) Compromise.

The principle of compromise/negotiation/mediation means that you find a middle ground with people you do not completely agree with. That way, you make your point known and also still protect the relationship you have with the other person involved. The other methods listed are not effective in resolving conflicts.

147. (D) She is protected by the Americans with Disabilities Act.

The Americans with Disabilities Act is a civil law that prohibits discrimination based on disability. Furthermore, this act entrusts employers with the responsibility of providing accommodations for employees with disabilities.

148. (A) Verbal appraisals are more useful than written appraisals.

This statement is incorrect because although verbal appraisals can be substituted for written reports, they are not more useful. You must give both verbal and written appraisals in a formal and standardized pattern.

149. (B) Subjective data is collected.

Informal appraisals are not objective assessments of a person's performance. Although they allow you to observe a person's performance in a natural setting and provide opportunities for collaboration and confrontation, they do not provide insight into the long-term performance of staff.

150. (A) Centralized.

In the centralized setting of the organization, information, including instructions and feedback, flows from top to bottom.

CPSIA information can be obtained
at www.ICGtesting.com
Printed in the USA
LVHW011946200521
688042LV00002B/18